Katrina's Recovery from Mysterious Disease

Kiss your Lyme, CFS,
Fibromyalgia and other
"Invisible" Illnesses Good-Bye

Katrina Starzhynskaya
Copyright © 2012 Health Mastery Publishing, INC

This book is not intended to provide medical advice or to take the place of medical advice and treatment from the reader's physician. Readers are advised to consult their own physicians or other qualified health professionals regarding treatments of their medical problems. Neither the publisher nor the author takes any responsibility for any possible consequences from any treatment, action or application of medicine, supplement, herb or preparation to any person reading or following the information in this book. If readers are taking prescription medications, they should consult with their physicians and not take themselves off of medicines without the proper supervision of a physician. If the reader has any questions concerning the information presented in this book, or its application to his or her particular medical profile, he or she should consult with his or her physician.

ISBN 978-0-9858118-0-8

ISBN-10: 0985811803

ISBN-13: 978-0-9858118-0-8

Dedication:

This book is dedicated to my mom Natalia and my dad Valeriy.

I left my home country at the age of 17 to pursue my dreams and goals.

While I've achieved success in all areas of my life, I feel the lack of family time spent together with my parents.

I want to let my mom and my dad know how much I love them.

Praise for
"Katrina's Recovery from Mysterious Disease".

"I highly encourage you to read this book full of options for body mind and spirit. There are treatment options in this book that I never even heard of and I am grateful that one person was courageous enough to bring these therapies forward so that others can learn -- patients and doctors alike."

Dr. Dan C. Rusu, M.D.

" This is a must-read if you are looking for serious inspiration and motivation to reclaim your life and not just survive but THRIVE. "

Meghan Snell

" I wish I had read this book years ago. It is easy to understand for EVERYONE, from the patient to the medical professional. You probably will NEVER be ill again if you read this book AND take actions! Exceptional!

Dr. Georgina Smith, PhD

"This book is the best guide to outstanding health–tells you exactly how to improve your health and go beyond; how to fight any and all sickness from lack of energy to Lyme Disease, CFS, Cancer, to name a few..."

Peter Crow

"Katrina's story of falling victim to an invisible illness and her journey towards possessing radiant health is not only mind empowering, she also helps shine a light on our own innate power of self-healing. You don't need to have Lyme disease to be inspired and benefit from this excellent book."

Dr. Laisan Leung L.Ac.

"*Katrina Starzhynskaya offers not just hope but practical solutions for all those who are battling chronic Lyme disease, Fibromyalgia, Chronic Fatigue Syndrome, and other degenerative illnesses and haven't had much help from the medical establishment.*"

Melissa K.

"*This is the best book I have ever read. I have been on many drugs and have seen many specialists, yet each year my health problems grew worse. When I got this book, I had no idea how it would change my life. Only six weeks after putting its suggestions to work, I am now off of all drugs and feeling better than I have in six years!*"

Nadia P.

"*This is probably the BEST book on health, bar none. It explains in very simple and easy to read terms how to reverse any degenerative disease and achieve outstanding health.*"

Mark G.

"*After losing a job due to chronic mysterious illness and being sick for 5 years I finally reclaimed my life back after following all the steps in this book.*

I wish doctors would have told me about these life changing therapies!"

James R.

"*A must read for all ages. This book is loaded with practical guides on how to reverse and/or prevent any dis-ease and stay healthy.*"

Ariel M.

Contents

1 What this Book is About and What You Need
to Know Before You Begin. x

Part 1   My Journey

2 What Made Me Write this Book
Lyme Disease Conference 17

3 Who am I?. 21

4 Montreal, mon épargnant... 27

5 It is ALL in YOUR HEAD!. 31

6 Dr. Raxlen, my first LLMD 39

7 Symptoms I Developed Due to Lyme. 41

8 What is Lyme disease? 45

9 Does Chronic Lyme Even Exist?. 49

10 Is Lyme disease a Biological Warfare?. 51

11 Welcome to the Club!
Now you are one of us, labeled "incurable"
Online Support Forums 57

12 Taking Full Responsibility for your Health. 61

13 Medical Prognosis. 65

14 Absolute Faith 69

15 Let's get straight to business...
Get rid of your story first and for good 73

16 A Look at Supplements
Antibiotics – Cure or Poison? 79

17 Cowden Protocol. 83

18 Artemisinin for Babesia 85

19 Date at the IV Room, Nutritional IVs. 87

20 Buhner's Protocol 91

21 Ondamed: The Wonder Device. .95

22 Acupuncture 97

23 Dr. Zhang and Modern Chinese Medicine 99

24 Two Feathers Healing Formula. 101

25 Acupuncture plus Apitherapy .105

26 Dr. Whitmont, Homeopathy 109

27 Derealization 111

28 Autohemotherapy. 113

29 Advanced Cell Training. 115

30 My Experience with a Rife Machine. 121

31 MMS – Miracle Mineral Solution 125

32 "Gu Syndrome" - Demons of the Body & Mind. 127

33 Chemtrails: What in the world are they spraying? 129

34 Brain Fog and How to Deal with It. 135

35 Family/ Friends Drama 141

36 Letters from those with "Invisible" Illnesses 149

37 Success Stories: Heather Levine, Marissa Cassella. 159

38 Mindset to Achieve Outstanding Health. 175

Part 2 Master Principles of Vibrant Health

1 Your Immune System is Your Best Doctor!. 183

2 Diet Equals Health!. 191

3 Gerson Therapy. 195

4 Body Cleansing 199

5 Bowel Cleanse 203

6 Parasite Cleanse 211

7 Dental Clean Up
   Mercury Amalgams 215

8 Danger of Root Canals, Cavitations 221

9 Kidney Cleanse 227

10 Liver/Gallbladder Cleanse, Flush 231

11 Juice Fast 241

12 Hyperthermia 245

13 Hydrotherapy/Contrast Showers 249

14 Dry Skin Brushing 253

15 Oil Pulling Therapy 257

16 Heliotherapy 263

17 Stop Your Sugar Addiction NOW! 273

18 Rebounding 279

19 Yoga 281

20 Detox 283

21 Natural Environment 287

22 Positivity, Laughter Therapy .293

23 Spiritual Healing 295

24 Kundalini Awakening
   by Tamara Balsamides 297

25 Final Thoughts 309

26 Acknowledgements 310

27 Notes 311

Keep in mind that no disease is impossible to cure. For the forces of nature, the rejuvenating capacity of constructive thoughts, and the healing power of faith and prayer, will support anyone who determines to become well.

Dr Gurudath

What this Book is About and What You Need to Know Before You Begin

❝You must know that in any moment a decision you make can change the course of your life forever: the very next person stand behind in line or sit next to on an airplane, the very next phone call you make or receive, the very next movie you see or book you read or page you turn could be the one single thing that causes the floodgates to open, and all of the things that you've been waiting for

to fall into place. **❞**

Anthony Robbins

Am I in the middle of a nightmare? Is this really happening to me? What happened to my life? Is my life really over? How do the doctors not know what's wrong with me? Does no one around me understand? I am so scared. I have tried hundreds of treatments and supplements and I am not any better. I have spent all my money on doctors and I am just getting worse. Won't someone please help me!?

Most days you have extreme fatigue and most nights you have insomnia. You wake up like you have not slept at all. You experience sharp stabbing headaches, excruciating joint pain, and you're barely able to cope with work or school because your brain feels so foggy that you forget how to perform simple tasks.

On some days, unpredictably, you have to miss school or work because your symptoms are multiplied. Migraines, random body aches, indigestion, neurological issues, joint and muscle pain, debilitating brain fog, fatigue, anxiety, depression, derealization - just to name a few. And no one really can see them and understand them. Five of six doctors told you that all your symptoms were psychological and it was *all in your head*, and the other one was baffled because your blood work and all medical tests known to mankind are "normal".

Your boss has told you that your job is at risk because you have taken too many sick days, and your family and friends think you are either making excuses or over-dramatizing your problems to avoid work and home chores and pretending to be sick for attention. *"But you look so good,"* they tell you. Abandoned by the closest and dearest people to you, you slowly lose hope and faith, you doubt if it's worth living like that, you are praying to God to either heal you or take you.

A few months or even years later you are diagnosed with Lyme, Fibromyalgia, CFS/ME or any other "invisible" illness.

And your journey begins…

When you're first diagnosed a warm feeling of peace washes over you. Now you have a "label" to put on your condition. Finally you know what is wrong with you and you are going to "take care" of it.

Then shock and denial sets in. You do some research about your diagnosis and realize it can be a death sentence. So you deny the reality of the diagnosis at some point in order to avoid emotional pain. Shock provides psychological protection from being overwhelmed all at once.

Then the anger at losing the life you once had overpowers you. You may rail against fate, questioning "Why me?" "What did I do wrong?"

Eventually the anger subsides and deep depression, anxiety and loneliness set in. Just when your friends and family may think you should be getting on with your life, a long period of sad reflection most likely overtakes you.

Does any of this sound familiar?

This book is an urgent warning for everyone. I know what it's like to live in this nightmare and worse. Believe me, it has been a long road to where I am today with my health and my life. I have denied, cried, pounded my head against the wall... and on my best days I've picked myself up yet again only to lose control over my life a few days later. I know what it's like to live for many years with pains, fatigue and brain fog. Many times, I've just wanted to give up. But I have also figured out how to conquer that noise in the back of my head that held me back and told me I would never be healthy again.

Chronic pains and physical suffering, anxiety and depression, depersonalization and derealization, extreme fatigue and brain fog, memory loss and confusion are very hard to suffer through because no one can relate and understand. I know how abandoned, isolated and detached they can make you feel. For most, they instigate a total catastrophe in your life causing you to separate from your loved ones, lose relationships, end your career, and generally cause you to be stagnant or debilitated in your life.

This book is not meant to be medical advice, but rather a personal account of my story; hopefully giving you some insight and confidence that there is a way to overcome debilitating chronic disease. However, I truly believe that if you apply all of the master principles of a vital life I discuss in Part 2 of this book, like your life depends on it (and it does!), you will recover from any degenerative illness in under a year. I hope that ultimately this book will teach you ways of reversing an invisible illness and help you to get your life back.

Furthermore, this book is not meant to provide information on the basics of Lyme disease, such as what it is, what the symptoms are, how it is contracted, what the standard treatments are and so forth.

This book is meant to inspire and empower you with my personal story along with some other success stories I have compiled. Also this book is for the family members of those who are currently battling Lyme disease, Chronic Fatigue Syndrome, Fibromyalgia and other "invisible" illnesses. It will help to open your eyes and hopefully your mind to really understand what your loved one is going through.

I know that many of us are alone, with no one in our lives we can vent to about our illness. Many of us are also desperate for any meaningful relief. Your doctor is supposed to understand and help you, right?

What I learned is that it is important, as with any "invisible" chronic illness, to FIRST work on your mindset to achieve a faster and more complete recovery. The reason is that your mind and your emotional health are going to be your foundation to get you through the scary aspects of healing the physical body.

Illness, most of the time, is caused by a weakened immune system due to chronic stress, poor diet, lack of exercise, and other stressors. This is why it is so important to restore your immune system first, while addressing the disruption, caused by a bacterial, viral or fungal infection, as well as environmental toxicity.

Let me offer my support and guide you through major steps for your recovery. Like many, I tried every possible treatment for Lyme with little improvement. Why? Because soon I realized that it was all about addressing my mental attitude, radically changing my life style, and supporting the immune system first instead of desperately seeking a cure.

How you handle the next step will determine how the rest of your life will be lived. You can try to focus on the positive aspects such as the things you're still able to do and the people who are there to support you, or you can be depressed and angry the rest of your life. It is your choice, my friend. I am here to help. Do not allow the disease to win the battle!

Part 1

My Journey

What Made Me Write this Book

LYME DISEASE CONFERENCE

"My greatest challenge has been to change the
mindset of people. Mindsets play strange tricks on
us. We see things the way our minds have instructed
our eyes to see. **"**

Muhammad Yunus

I am sitting here, at the Lyme disease conference in
San Diego, CA May 6, 2012, presented by Dr. Richard
Horowitz, one of the most knowledgeable Lyme literate
doctors in the world!

There are people with their IV's, some are barely moving with walkers, some are just looking and feeling exhausted and sick. Some wearing sunglasses due to light
sensitivity, many wear earplugs due to sound sensitivity
(or both).

The first speaker was Brooke Landau, the former high-
fashion runway model and current weathercaster for a
local TV news station in San Diego. Brooke had an amazing future in front of her; she graduated from college and

was embarking on a career as an international marketing manager with a Fortune 500 company. Then a bite from a bug no bigger than a poppy seed changed all that. Her life was put on hold as she spent the next seventeen years battling a disease that almost cost Landau her life.

Brooke encouraged the audience to have hope and patience, because that was the only resort left for Lyme sufferers.

I was thinking how lucky and grateful I was to be healthy again, to be healed, to be FREE of Lyme disease! The girl sitting next to me was crying during Brooke's speech. The guy next to me was popping pills during the presentation; the whole crowd looked so exhausted, tortured, and distressed. I could feel the pain and agony these people were going through, because I went through this hell myself!

During the break the majority of the audience went to Starbucks®, including myself. I was observing everyone and thanking God I was over the pain that Lyme brings.

People were ordering lattes, mochas, with double espresso and triple caramel sauce and whipped cream; pairing coffee with muffins, brownies, cupcakes and other sweets - even worse some were adding artificial sweeteners to their coffee.

Only two people ordered a cup of tea and grabbed an apple... myself and the older lady that looked pretty healthy.

After the break, the conference continued with a Q&A session.

Some of the questions:

How to make insurance pay for the treatments?

What antibiotics to take and in what order?

Will drug X cure me?

Not one person asked, *"What can I do to assist my body in healing? What lifestyle changes should I address? What diet should I be on?"*

Everyone was looking for a "cure". Everyone wanted to delegate responsibility for his or her own health to someone else. And I completely understand; I've been there. At one time, I had been looking for a "cure" as well.

The whole business of medicine brainwashes us in to believing that we need to focus on "finding a cure". The word "finding" in itself implies having to look outside of one's own self.

That day I realized what made me different from the crowd; I got insight as to why I was able to overcome a so called "incurable" disease and why so many people are still suffering.

When I was extremely sick I thought if I ever recover, I am going to write a book to help others. However after my recovery I moved on with my life and I had no time for a book. I was too busy making a living to pay off my "Lyme" debt. At the conference, I was so broken up by witnessing the suffering of those who are still battling Lyme that I made a promise to myself to write this book and get my message out to those who need it most.

Who am I?

66The part can never be well unless the whole is well. 99

Plato

Well, hello there.

My name is Katrina Starzhynskaya and I am originally from Minsk, Belarus. I have always been ambitious in my life so after graduating from high school I decided to move to the U.S.A. to pursue my career.

I came to the United States in 1998 with $500 in my pocket, a small suitcase, and I only knew one friend who lived in New York City. Back then I did not realize the many obstacles I would have to overcome to make it to where I am today. I had no papers, no work authorization, and my English was very weak.

I graduated from Baruch Business School, and then started my master's degree in Oriental Medicine. I then went on to start my own business and I became a successful entrepreneur in the health and wellness industry. I enjoyed playing tennis, working out, teaching yoga, and modeling. I just loved life!

Also, I was a total health fanatic. My diet was super healthy (or so I thought at that time). I was going on periodic juice or water fasts, exercising, meditating; you name it. I hadn't had a common cold or flu since I was 10 years old. Overall, I enjoyed great physical health.

October 29, 2009 — my life turned upside down...

The night before, I had gone to sleep planning my next day — French lessons, medical school, clients, and yoga. I was envisioning my bright future in front of me - happy, healthy and vibrant. Little did I know what life had planned for me...

I woke up in horrible pain. My limbs were numb, half of my face was paralyzed, and my head was in agony... and this was just scratching the surface; I really can't begin to describe all the horror I felt.

I ended up at the NYU ER, in New York City. After waiting about 4 hours in line, some intern looked at me and diagnosed me with Bell's palsy. Then finally an MD showed up and diagnosed me with an "idiopathic" condition, which means no known cause and no cure. No tests were done at all! None! She prescribed me steroids and antivirals and sent me home! I asked the doctor if I should do acupuncture to help me with Bell's palsy, at which she replied, "ACUPUNCTURE - oh NO, don't do that! Don't let them touch your face!" What an ignorant doctor, she just left me half paralyzed with no proactive suggestions.... I was treated so inhumanely by hospital employees; all they cared about was my insurance card.

The whole day I was traveling from one hospital to the next and finding no answers. Even knowing it was an emergency, they told me to bring two referrals and that the next available appointment would be two months from that day!

My last stop was my acupuncture school in the city.

What a contrast between western medical doctors and healers! I got to see a doctor right away plus I had two more interns working on me. I was treated with so much compassion and care. There is something I want to share with you guys – I had asked a doctor if I should take steroids, and his answer was, *"Well, I can tell you one thing – if you take them or if you do not, you'll get the same result either way."* My point is that the doctors are so scared of being sued, that they can't really express their own personal opinions. And being in acupuncture school for four years, I was really disappointed to find out that it is out of our scope of practice to give any medical advice if we do not want to get sued! The moral of this particular story is: YOU, not your doctor, not your healer, but you have to make the ultimate decisions about what medical approach you are going to take.

I continued going back for my acupuncture treatments every single day for five days in a row; however I did not see any results. I was losing hope. Now I know that five days was not necessarily a lot, but I was desperate.

I was really scared and was feeling so alone. I was not able to tell my parents because I had no idea what was wrong with me. Plus, they were overseas so they would not be able to help me anyway.

My days became so different... I literally lost control over my life.

I started having major panic attacks. The fear and sorrow inside me made me insane. The only hope I had was to receive emotional support from my sister and her husband, but they were not there for me and did not seem to care.

I was in my small Manhattan apartment all by myself in complete darkness (because I had already developed light sensitivity and it hurt terribly to see myself in the mirror disabled with a half paralyzed face) with only a candle lit, I burned some incense and lavender to tranquilize my mind. Tears would constantly break through and I would go from total numbness to a state of panic....

I was either in a comatose state or online desperately looking for a solution. It was crucial that I found a solution in a timely manner because if I did not restore facial muscle movement within a short period of time—I may never be able to blink my eye or to smile again! That was frightening!

I was blessed to meet a total stranger online who helped me through. Dr. Peter Veniez a holistic doctor, hypnotherapist, and coach, put me under hypnosis via Skype to withdraw me from shock and fear. He encouraged me to come to Montreal to get treatments from a Chinese healer he knew.

As soon as I heard about the healer I decided to go. I was so sick; I thought I would not even be able to get there by myself. I very much needed someone to go with me. I have never in my life asked anyone for help. I have always been "Miss Independent". Remember, I came to this country under the age of 18 with $500 in my pocket and had to figure it all out on my own. I never asked anyone for money, shelter, etc. But now I was not able to take care of myself anymore. Something was going on with me, something was wrong; VERY wrong and I did not know what it was. It was very hard for me to admit and to set aside that "independent" side of me and start begging for help. I called my sister and other close people to ask for help. Unfortunately, everyone was busy with his or her own life. The only person who did not ask questions but just packed and went with me was my friend Olga (I am really grateful to her even though she had no driver's license; just her moral support was comforting).

So, here I am, totally sick, having tidal fevers, emotional outbursts, feeling constantly cold, in excruciating pain, and having numbness in my limbs driving myself to Montreal. Yes, my limbs were getting numb and I had to manage driving manual transmission. I was unable to blink my left eye so it would constantly dry out, therefore I could not really see properly. I have to admit, I am a speed addict. I cannot drive slowly; just can't. Sports cars and speed are my biggest addiction. Even when I was that sick, I managed to drive even faster than I usually do, I really wanted to make it to Montreal as quickly as possible, and I was already driving for 10 hours straight. It was an extremely dark November night; no cars, no lights, no nothing! I was having a really hard time concentrating on the road. All of a sudden I saw a "disco" light in my rear view mirror. Sure enough, I got pulled over. I could really care less; what was a speeding ticket when my life was on a cliff? Yes, I got a speeding ticket and 8 points!

When we reached the border, the officer asked us where we were heading to and he wanted to see some kind of papers. Of course, I did not have any itinerary, I booked my hotel, however did not print the confirmation, and other than that I did not have any papers. So border officials kept us for a couple of hours at the border while they were checking our final destination.

I had not taken a road trip forever; I thought this would be a nice therapy and would distract my mind from my trauma... BUT I was WRONG. I was so broken down that I was praying just to make it there to Montreal in one piece. I am grateful to my friend Brigitta who checked on me regularly. She was the only person who called me to make sure I arrived. Yes, my sister or other people close to me at the time who knew how sick I was never even called to check on me.

Montreal, mon épargnant...

Dr. Peter picked me up from my hotel with his beautiful wife Brigitte and took me to Ceciline, the healer. I call the sessions I had with Ceciline, "Chinese torture". Yes, the kind of torture you see in horror movies. And being an acupuncture student at that time, I had an idea how needles felt – and well, they were nothing like Ceciline's! I was getting close to a 100 needles on my front side – my legs, arms, stomach, ears and face. (There are 361 acupuncture points on the classical meridians and hundreds of additional acupuncture points. More points are being discovered each year). She was not gentle at all with her insertion technique, and she was pretty rough with manipulating the needles. So after she was done with her technique, her husband would come in and give me a "foot rub". Don't get too excited! That was the worst "Chinese torture" I had ever experienced. And my pain threshold is very high. I never take any painkillers and I ask for 1/8 of an average dental anesthesia for major procedures. (My friend Olga heard me screaming from outside the building). Ceciline's husband, from what I thought, was trying to break my foot bones – he was twisting and pulling them so hard; I was crying and screaming. This particular procedure *is* a traditional Chinese technique to restore nerve function. And I was up for any torture; I desperately wanted my face control back more than anything else! With losing my face, I lost my life! I lost my business, modeling jobs, friends, and dates - my livelihood! I had no idea how I would survive financially because I had started spending my savings already and it costs a lot of money for medical procedures!

After he was done, I would flip over and get over 100 needles on my back, including my scalp. Then Ceciline's assistant would come in and she would perform cupping and bleeding on me. The whole treatment took anywhere between 3 to 4 hours, with three people working on me, and Ceciline charged me $50 bucks! Yes, $50 bucks! In the U.S. a doctor would not even talk to you for $50 bucks!

After a couple of treatments she told me, *"I will not charge you anymore, I just want to help you."* Moreover, she graciously allowed me to stay as long as I needed to at her sisters hotel - for almost no cost.

After her treatments Dr. Peter took me to his clinic for more hypnotherapy sessions to help me recuperate and get better (I just want to make it clear, Dr. Peter Veniez had never asked me to pay him and had insisted on helping me from the bottom of his heart) . I HAVE NEVER MET SUCH WONDERFUL PEOPLE BEFORE! God Bless them!

And screw you; a medical doctor from NYU emergency room – that arrogant young woman who did not test me for anything (they did not even take my temperature), never mentioned any possibility of any infectious disease, told me to NEVER get acupuncture, prescribed steroids (steroids can actually kill someone with encephalitis – brain inflammation due to Lyme) and sent me a bill for over $1, 000! If I were tested for Lyme that day, in the emergency room, my life would be completely different. I would not have gone through over two years of pure hell and desperation.

I made it back to NYC after a week of recovering and I was so full of hope. My facial muscles started responding in about a week; in 10 days I was able to semi-smile. In about two weeks no one could tell I had just previously been paralyzed. Those two weeks helped me grow tremendously. I reevaluated my life, my friends, my family, and my VALUES. What mattered two weeks prior, did not mean anything now. I knew how precious life is and had a new appreciation for things that we usually take for granted. I did not feel great, but I had my face back and it gave me hope! I was experiencing extreme fatigue, weakness, aches and pains, neurological problems like twitches and nerve shootings. I had all kinds of weird sensations like something was crawling all over my body. Sometimes I felt like I had wet spots on my legs; other times there were burning sensations like someone was twisting my arm out. Something was going on constantly! 24/7! But I was happy I was recovering, so I tried not to worry. Little did I know that it was just the beginning of my "journey"....

It is all in Your Head!

Upon returning to New York, I resumed school and continued with acupuncture treatments. The practitioners were amazing and were taking good care of me. However, I had learned another lesson while one of the practitioners was doing the usual "intake", meaning asking me all kinds of health questions. She asked me how my diet was. I told her I was a vegetarian. So she looked at me with a smile and told me, *"Maybe you can add filet mignon at least once a week. You are blood deficient and that could be the cause of your facial paralysis."* (Blood deficiency in TCM does not mean anemia). Well, at that stage of my life, I would agree to eat not only a piece of flesh; I would eat *anything* that, although I considered disgusting, suggested the possibility to help me to heal and avoid future paralysis! However, something told me she was wrong! First of all, that woman was over 300 pounds, so she was not a role model for me. Second – my intuition told me that my illness had nothing to do with eating a freakin' filet mignon! And I am glad I did not listen to her and never touched meat!

In a couple of days, I had another acupuncture treatment and the intern while needling me was telling me, *"Be careful now, because if you had facial paralysis, it will only get worse. So if you do not make changes, you can become paralyzed again. And all diet sodas and artificial sweeteners are horrible for you; they cause all kinds of neurological dysfunctions."* I was about to run from the table! How can a healer use scarcity and pure non-sense with the patient? First off, I never even touched any soda, and I never use any artificial sweeteners! The point is some medical doctors, as well as healers, can be ignorant and simply boneheaded. Always listen to your intuition and use your common sense!

Six weeks later I became even sicker than before. All my pains tripled; neurological problems progressed, facial muscle twitches moved from my left side to the right. I became so paranoid that my right side was going to become paralyzed. I had no idea what was going on with me, I was so scared. I lost my mind and total control over my life. I started experiencing heart palpitations and really bad panic attacks. I was waking up at night in a cold sweat. In fact, the night sweats were so bad, I had to change my pajamas twice a night; they were soaking wet. During those panic attacks I thought I was dying while desperately gasping for air. I cannot fully explain how I felt! I was trying to describe some of it to my sister; she would reply that it was all in my head! Then doctors would tell me it was ALL IN MY HEAD! I was beyond scared and terrified! All by myself, all alone in this country, not a single soul seemed to care, not a single soul showed a sign of compassion... that was the beginning of the hardest period of my life. I knew I was not crazy, but I was in constant pain; pain that was constantly migrating from place to place and I was experiencing weird sensations all over my body, but everyone told me it was ALL IN MY HEAD! I was so desperate; I was crying my heart out 24/7 not knowing what was wrong with me and what to do about that fact!

Ninety days after waking up partially paralyzed, I woke up with something even more "wrong" than before.

And I had a feeling something bad was coming my way. I got dressed and drove to New Jersey to see another acupuncturist. I was a total mess. My eyes were black from so many needles I had taken in the past three months and red and swollen from crying. I lost a lot of weight (first I was not able to eat due to my half-paralyzed face, and then I had no appetite). I was crying my heart out at another doctor's office begging for help, asking what was wrong with me. She told me I had "wind" in my body. Yes, I knew that I had "wind", but what was causing it? What freakin' demons possessed my body and my head???

I left her office and while walking to my car I saw "normal" people going out, shopping, going to the gym, or jogging. They all seemed so happy and carefree. I was not "normal" anymore. Something possessed my body, something was SO WRONG, and no one seemed to understand, and that was scary! I got into my car and made a phone call – for the first time in my life I called my sister's in-laws and asked if I could stay over at their house in Morristown, NJ. I had a feeling something bad was coming and I was losing my mind. I needed to be around people so someone could call an ambulance when this "something bad" arrived. Well, that "something bad" did not make us wait too long.

I was rushed by ambulance to Morristown ER. Everybody thought I was having a stroke because the left side of my body became totally numb, my blood pressure dropped, and I was only half conscious. At that moment, I felt so at peace for the first time in the previous three months – I thought: if I was dying at least I was not by myself in my small Manhattan apartment and if it was not my time yet, I was in an emergency room and they will do what they can.

I was hooked up to an IV right away and soon after, I was rolled away for every kind of test possible: CT scan,

MRI's, X-rays, blood tests, and some others of which I had no idea what they actually were. For one of the CT scans I was given an IV with a contrast dye and then put immediately into some capsule that closed completely once my body was inside of it. Besides feeling like a monkey in a research lab, I got sick from the dye and had a major panic attack from being in a closed space. After they got me out I was immediately given another IV to stop an allergic reaction from the dye and I was injected with a sedative. I felt like a small tortured rat undergoing medical experiments. My life was more hellish than it already was and the emergency room experience made it even worse. After 12 hours of testing nothing was found to be wrong with me and I was pronounced "healthy" and free to go home. It was my second ER visit to one of the best hospitals in the country and according to the doctors NOTHING WAS WRONG with me - again!

Before I left, a resident told me I should see a neurologist and gave me a referral.

December 23, 2009. Yes, right before Christmas I walked into The Neuroscience Center of Northern New Jersey with my referral but without an appointment; I just went directly there.

Of course I was told that Dr. Fox was fully booked and I should check back after Christmas. I could not afford to take "No" for an answer. I decided I was going to sit there and wait in case someone did not show up or worst-case, I would beg a doctor to see me after his final patient. I arrived at the clinic in the morning and while I was patiently waiting… what I saw was a very devastating picture – people in wheelchairs, with all kinds of neurological problems; I was really scared I could end up like one of them. Every half hour I would bug a receptionist to see if by any chance someone had cancelled or did not show up. Right before lunch time I was back by the front desk checking if I had any possibility of seeing a neurologist. I was lucky enough that some doctor was leaving for lunch and heard me desperately begging the receptionist to squeeze me in. I am really grateful to Matthew Frank Conigliari, M.D., who agreed to see me during his lunch-time without an appointment. The doctor took off his coat and invited me to his office. First, he was asking me some weird questions like what date it was. And you know what? At the time – I had no idea what date it was; I could care less! All I knew was that I was really sick but I was NOT crazy! That was my lucky day I guess – I was sitting in the office of not just a compassionate person, but a very smart doctor. After all kinds of neurological tests, and finding nothing wrong with me again, he finally announced, *"You are not crazy, you have Lyme disease!"* My reaction was, *"Lyme what?"* I have never heard of that disease before (being an acupuncture student). He explained to me what Lyme disease was and told me to start antibiotics RIGHT AWAY!

On my way home, I was super excited and happy! Yes, you got me right – happy! I thought to myself, "Finally I know what's wrong with me and I am going to take care of it!" Well, my excitement lasted for about 10 minutes till I reached my sister's in-laws house. As soon as I got in, I Googled "Lyme" and realized -- I had a long road ahead of me...

Those who know me know that I never take any pharmaceutical drugs; NEVER - period. Well, not this time! I went to fill my prescription right away! After researching Lyme disease for only an hour and realizing that I was experiencing all the corresponding symptoms, I would take not just drugs; I would eat horse poop if it could heal me. Many legitimate sources online were stating that Lyme was worse than cancer, AIDS and all kinds of degenerative diseases combined!

The next day my sister and her in-laws were flying to Mexico for Christmas and New Year's. They go for a family vacation every Christmas to celebrate. I was invited before, but I always refused; preferring to stay in the city with my friends and go out. This time I was not able to stay in the city on my own - who would call an ambulance next time I get sick?

Every time I am flying somewhere I get really excited– I just love the energy of the airport. Despite it being hectic, it's moving, never stagnate - it feels full of promising changes in your life. Well, this time it was DIFFERENT... I was like a zombie walking to our gate; looking at people and thinking how lucky they were – they were healthy and all their problems were NOTHING compared to mine! I was just 28 years old, full of ambitions, hopes, dreams and goals. And all of these dreams crashed yesterday when I found out just how ill I really was - terribly ill with a "mysterious" and "incurable" disease. My mind was half numb, I could not take the emotional turmoil anymore; I did not care if the plane I was getting on crashed.

While in Mexico I was desperately researching Lyme and calling all LLMD (Lyme Literate Medical Doctors) offices to sign up. Yes, sign up. With Lyme disease it's like you become a member of that suffering community, you visit doctors and experiment with drugs and treatments for the rest of your life. I was reading reviews and was getting more and more depressed. For example, one of the LLMDs from somewhere in NJ was the "best" according to some forum, because apparently she had chronic Lyme disease, as well as, both of her kids so, "she knew best how to treat it." Another review was for a doctor in upstate New York. He specialized in infectious diseases and, "when you wait in line, you sit next to terminally ill AIDS patients." Moreover, 90% of LLMDs did not take new patients anymore, because they are fully booked and they had been harassed by insurance companies and legal agencies. (The reason for that, I'll cover in another chapter). The other 10% had a 6 to 12 month waiting list. 6 to 12 months!!! I became mentally paralyzed, terrified, scared, and depressed! If a doctor was not able to heal her own kids and herself—Lyme is no freakin' joke! There is NO CURE! Will I still be alive in 6 months? What am I to do? And of course they do not accept any insurance, because simply no insurance company covers Lyme disease treatments. An appointment to see a LLMD on average is between $800 to $1,200 plus the cost of blood tests!

"Based on my personal experience, I estimate that 90% of primary care physicians and family doctors have no idea what they are doing concerning diagnosis and treatment of tickborne disease. They will probably look at you like you are crazy, misdiagnose and under treat you, not treat you at all, or try to send you to a shrink. Lyme disease is everywhere! It is very serious and it is spreading all over the world."

- Laura W.

"Most of my HIV patients used to die... now most don't ... Some still do, of course. My Lyme patients, the sickest ones, want to die but they can't. That's right, they want to die but they can't. The most common cause of death in Lyme disease is suicide. In the current day, if one compares HIV/AIDS to Lyme Borreliosis Complex patients in issues of 1) access to care, 2) current level of science, and 3) the levels of acceptance by doctors and the public, patients suffering with advanced Lyme Borreliosis Complex have an inferior quality of life compared to those with HIV/AIDS...."

- Dr. Jemsek

Dr. Raxlen, my first LLMD

66If you don't take care of your body, where are you going to live? 99

Unknown

Finally, I secured an appointment with Carolyn Welcome, PA in Dr. Raxlen's office in New York City. Dr. Raxlen had a waiting list of about 6 months, so I got to see his PA. Carolyn was really nice, caring, and knowledgeable. At last - I felt like someone knew exactly what was going on with me because when I was explaining to her about my weird sensations, unlike all the other doctors, she knew exactly what I was talking about and even had names for them. After taking down my medical history, Carolyn muscle tested me. I was holding different containers next to my thymus gland. My hand remained strong to containers with HIV, cancer virus and all other microorganisms that were there. Alas, my hand became extremely weak and went down. I read the label on a container I was holding at the moment: "borrelia burgdorferi" (bug that causes Lyme disease).

Carolyn gave me information about Dr. Zhang, and

really encouraged me to go see him. She also told me about the device called, 'Ondamed' and gave me a whole list of natural supplements to take. The list was close to 30 different ones, including Samento, Artemisia, different herbs, vitamins, omega oils, colloidal silver, and other good stuff.

Carolyn was always available by e-mail to answer any questions. She always got back to me within 24 hours every time I had questions and concerns and she took her time to explain all the little details I was inquiring about.

I am really grateful to Dr. Raxlen and Carolyn for their help and dedication to their patients.

Three weeks later my Western blot results came in, I had 2 bands positive and 2 unidentified. That was my "official" diagnose with Lyme disease.

Symptoms I Developed Due to Lyme

Head, Face, Neck
- Headache, mild or severe
- Pressure in head
- Twitching of facial or other muscles
- Facial paralysis (Bell's Palsy)
- Tingling of nose, (tip of) tongue, cheek
- Stiff or painful neck
- Jaw pain or stiffness (TMJ)
- Dental problems (unexplained), toothaches
- Sore throat, runny nose

Eyes/Vision
- Double or blurry vision
- Increased floating spots
- Pain in eyes, or swelling around eyes
- Oversensitivity to light

Ears/Hearing
- Buzzing in ears

- Pain in ears
- Oversensitivity to sounds
- Ringing in one or both ears

Digestive and Excretory Systems

- Constipation
- Irritable bladder
- Upset stomach (nausea or pain)

Musculoskeletal System

- Bone pain, joint pain or swelling, carpal tunnel syndrome
- Stiffness of joints, back, neck, tennis elbow
- Muscle pain or cramps, (Fibromyalgia)

Respiratory and Circulatory Systems

- Shortness of breath, can't get full/satisfying breath
- Chest pain or rib soreness
- Night sweats or unexplained chills
- Heart palpitations or extra beats

Neurological System

- Burning or stabbing sensations in the body
- Fatigue, Chronic Fatigue Syndrome
- Weakness, peripheral neuropathy
- Pressure in the head
- Numbness in body, tingling, pinpricks
- Dizziness
- Lightheadedness, wooziness

Psychological well-being

- Mood swings, irritability

- Unusual depression
- Disorientation (getting or feeling lost)
- De-realization
- Feeling as if you are losing your mind
- Overly-emotional reactions, crying easily
- Too much sleep, or insomnia
- Difficulty falling or staying asleep
- Panic attacks, anxiety

Mental Capability

- Memory loss (short or long term)
- Confusion, difficulty in thinking
- Difficulty with concentration or reading
- Going to the wrong place
- Forgetting how to perform simple tasks

General Well-being

- Extreme fatigue
- Swollen glands/lymph nodes
- Unexplained fevers (high or low grade)
- Symptoms seem to change; come and go
- Pain migrates (moves) to different body parts
- Early on, experienced a "flu-like" illness, after which you have not felt well since
- Low body temperature

Allergies/Chemical sensitivities

- Increased effect from processed foods and processed sugar.

And according to the doctors nothing was wrong with me; it was all in my head!

What is Lyme Disease?

"Having battled cancer, getting pneumonia 3 times, splitting my face wide open (horse accident - causing me to lose my voice for a year) now all seem like a 'cakewalk' compared to what I've experienced in the last couple of years. Waking up in the middle of the night with half of my body paralyzed (with the rest of it tingling) and my brain shutting down as if I were having a stroke was a terrifying experience. It was a lonely and scary ride in the ambulance and in the ER by myself. Little did I know then that I was about to enter into the 'twilight zone' of systemic diseases, which is turning out to be a very long and painful journey both physically and emotionally. To this day, I really don't know exactly when, how or where I contracted this nightmare – Lyme disease." Deanna B.

According to Dr. Scott Taylor, DVM one of the most brilliant scientists studying Lyme disease, Lyme is a seriously complex multi-system inflammatory disease that is triggered by the bacterial lipoproteins produced by the spiral-shaped bacteria called Borrelia. Borrelia is difficult to isolate, grow, and study in the laboratory. So, our technical knowledge of this pathogen is poor compared to our understanding of most bacteria that cause disease. Transmission of Borrelia occurs primarily through the bite of ticks. The disease affects every tissue and every major organ system in the body. Clinically, it can appear as a chronic arthralgia (joint pain), fibromyalgia (fibrous connective tissue and muscle pain), chronic fatigue, immune dysfunction and as a neurological disease. Lyme disease may even be fatal in severe cases.

The diagnosis of Lyme disease is primarily based upon clinical evidence. There is currently no laboratory test that is definitive for Lyme disease. Many tests give false negative results. Physicians not familiar with the complex clinical presentation of Lyme disease frequently misdiagnose it as other disorders such as: Fibromyalgia or Chronic Fatigue Immune Dysfunction Syndrome (CFIDS), Multiple Sclerosis, Lupus, Parkinson's, Alzheimer's, Rheumatoid Arthritis, Motor Neuron Disease (ALS, Amyotrophic Lateral Sclerosis -Lou Gehrig's disease), Multiple Chemical Sensitivity Syndrome (MCS) and numerous other psychiatric disorders such as depression and anxiety.

"Lyme disease is a familiar name to most people, but their knowledge of it is very limited. Unfortunately, this is also true for most professionals in the medical community. There have been numerous reports in the media about it in the United States over the past 25 years. These superficial articles report something about small deer ticks transmitting bacteria called Borrelia burgdorferi. The tick vectors are said to be mainly restricted to certain endemic areas of the United States, which are the Northeast and the upper Midwest. Frequently mentioned is the bulls-eye skin rash that develops following the bite of an infected tick. The disease is reported to begin with flu-like symptoms that progress to an arthritic and fibromyalgia-like condition. It is often said that Lyme disease can be readily treated with standard regimens of antibiotics. While these reports are partially true, they are also critically erroneous and very misleading!

Lyme disease is devastating the lives of hundreds of thousands of individuals and we are all at risk. Many patients are suffering with chronic Lyme disease and continue to be misdiagnosed and mistreated. In many cases of Lyme disease, a correct diagnosis doesn't occur until after several months or more often many years of suffering with the disease. By then it has caused severe illness, disability and permanent damage. The disease is widespread and the prevalence is significantly higher than reported by health officials."

Here is an interesting quote from Dr. Scott Taylor, DVM, *"It is very unfortunate that most physicians don't know how to recognize and treat cases of Lyme disease, especially the illusive cases of chronic Lyme disease. I'm not just talking about general MDs being ignorant; I am also referring to specialists such as: rheumatologists, neurologists, orthopedic surgeons, cardiologists, psychiatrists, and the most ignorant actually seem to be infectious disease specialists. I was extremely surprised by this plague of ignorance after I began my investigation of Lyme disease."*

Lyme disease is unlike any other syndrome on the planet. Alternative practitioners note that it is more difficult to treat than cancer. The reason for this is that it is a bioengineered, complex combination of thousands of viruses, parasites, fungi, mycoplasma, and other organisms. It is designed to be undetectable in the early stages, untreatable, and eventually, permanently disabling. It is also designed to get worse if treatment is attempted, a phenomenon observed in the Herxheimer reactions noted by those who try to treat their Lyme disease.

Does Chronic Lyme Even Exist?

There is a controversy surrounding Lyme disease, which has prevented most of the Lyme sufferers from being properly diagnosed and from being treated accordingly for the disease. The core of the dispute is persistence of infection versus autoimmunity.

One side of the medical institution stands up for the idea that Lyme disease is extremely hard to catch and very easy to cure. Its proponents promote short-term antibiotic treatment of just a few weeks that unfortunately do not do anything for those with Lyme disease. Nine out of ten patients not only remain very ill after that course of antibiotics, but also feel worse than before the treatment. When that happens with other diseases, patients are given longer courses of antibiotics until the infection is eradicated. However, proponents holding this viewpoint, including the IDSA (Infectious Diseases Society of America) and insurance companies   have taken strong actions to prevent Lyme patients from receiving any more antibiotics beyond the first few weeks of treatment. Their claim is any remaining symptoms, after the short course of antibiotics, are "autoimmune" in nature, not a persistent infection.

The other point of view is held by physicians who are

treating chronic Lyme patients, most Lyme Literate Medical Doctors. They insist that scientific research shows that even after longer term treatment that can be anywhere from 6 to 18 months or even more with antibiotics, most of the Lyme bacteria survive, which is called persistent infection. They also admit that although some symptoms can be the result of an autoimmune chaos, that chaos is driven by a load of Lyme bacteria and other co-infections (including Bartonella, Babesia, micoplasma, fungi, viruses) that persist after treatment. These groups of doctors and scientists have found that repeated courses of long term antibiotics, in some cases intravenous antibiotics, and combinations of antibiotics often help patients to regain some functionality. (However, I would like to note that most of LLMDs while treating Lyme patients with long-term antibiotics, add a long herbal protocol to boost their immune system and decrease the load of infection.)

Most of the Lyme advocates, patients, LLMDs and other physicians find that the standards for what the disease is, how it can be treated, how it can be tested for, and what science can be published on Lyme disease are highly censored and there is an "iron curtain" around Lyme disease.

Is Lyme Disease a Biological Warfare?

When the neurologist diagnosed me with Lyme disease based on clinical manifestation, he explained that it's an infectious disease and I needed to take a course of antibiotics. He warned me that I needed to be on Doxycycline for at least 90 days without any breaks. I got really concerned - why would I need to be on antibiotics for such a long period of time, when a standard course of antibiotics for infectious disease is 7-14 days? Little did I know that 90 days is nothing, usual Lyme treatment is 18 to 36 MONTHS of IV plus oral antibiotics with a slim chance of being cured.

Let me ask you something; how come an infectious disease like Pneumonia, for example, is treatable within 7-10 days of taking oral antibiotics, while an infectious disease like Lyme requires up to 36 MONTHS of intravenous antibiotics without any guarantees?

"Current recommendations call for 7 - 10 days of treatment for S. pneumoniae and 10 - 14 days for Mycoplasma pneumoniae and Chlamydia pneumoniae. However, some research suggests that patients with mild-to-moderate community-acquired pneumonia may be successfully treated with 7 days or less of antibiotics. The shorter treatment may increase patient tolerance, and improve the likelihood that patients will stick to

the treatment regimen. It will also help limit the growing problem of antibiotic resistance."

If I was not ill with Lyme, I would never be able to understand how it really feels. When I try to explain it, people think I am crazy. It is hard to even explain to a doctor what hurts, because the pain migrates before you finish your sentence. Pains due to Lyme are UNBEARABLE! I have never experienced anything like that before. It felt like someone was twisting my arm out, pain was coming through my bones. Joint pain was devastating. Headaches and migraines were terrifying!

But forget the physical pain! What was going on inside my brain was much worse! First off, I had constant muscle twitches, nerve shootings, I had weird sensations like bugs were crawling on me, like rain was coming down and I felt wet drops on my body. And all of that was not actually as bad as derealization! During really bad derealization moments, I wanted to kill myself. It was so scary to see the whole world around you in a different dimension. That sensation was terrifying: so much so that I was praying to God to either stop it or take me.

Being an acupuncture student, I have seen all kinds of patients in our New York City clinic. AIDS, cancer, MS, fibromyalgia, you name it –we got those patients. Trust me; none of them were as ill as Lyme patients. Even AIDS patients did not experience anything even close to derealization and depersonalization.

I can go on and on, but no need. What we are experiencing is not caused by some "natural" bug that the most potent herbs or antibiotics are able to kill. I have never heard of another infectious disease that causes this much physical pain and agony, neurological dysfunction, paralysis, mental dysfunctions, and the highest rate of suicide!

Just read a book called *Lab 257* by Michael C. Carroll.

Situated near the Hamptons, the posh playground and a weekend getaway from New York City; amongst the popular spot of celebrities and "trust fund" types, lies a mysterious island unidentified on most maps. On the few it can be found, Plum Island is marked red or yellow and stamped U. S. Government – restricted or dangerous animal disease. Despite its innocent name, Plum Island is an origin of some of the most dangerous and deadly viruses on the planet. From African swine flu and West Nile virus, to Rift Valley fever, Plum Island tests a host of deadly diseases.

Carroll's seven years of research of Plum Island compiled a compelling argument that the introduction of Lyme disease, West Nile virus, and other diseases may all have been "coincidental" releases from the island's lab. Carroll points out the apparent history of mismanagement and neglect, poor construction and faulty power lines, along with malfunctioning incinerators and vents which apparently do not contain a proper airflow. Mr. Carroll documents a list of problems that could have threatened the lives of millions.

Carroll's point is that scientists were working with the strains of viruses not native to North America; however outbreaks of each occurred just a few miles away from the island. A Lyme disease outbreak was recorded at Old Lyme, Connecticut, in a remarkable proximity to the island. The first reported case of West Nile virus was recorded near Plum Island as well.

Lab 257 exposes the secret world of a federal government germ laboratory. It presents frightening revelations including virus outbreaks, biological meltdowns, infected workers, periodic flushing of contaminated raw sewage into area waters, and the sneaky connection between Plum Island, Lyme disease, and the deadly 1999 West Nile virus outbreak.

FROM MY INBOX:

The existence of the Lyme disease epidemic is officially cov-
ered up in the UK, its myriad presentations routinely misdiag-
nosed as everything from "M.E." to MS to hypochondria. This
is the first admission by a US government body that the cause
is an incapacitating bio war agent:

'SAN ANTONIO (AP) -- The $10.6 million Margaret
Batts Tobin Laboratory Building will provide a 22,000-square-
foot facility to study such diseases as anthrax, tularemia, chol-
era, Lyme disease, desert valley fever and other parasitic and
fungal diseases. The Centers for Disease Control and Preven-
tion identified these diseases as potential bioterrorism agents.'

So, for the first time, a US government body admits that
Lyme disease is a biological warfare agent. This is the reason
that hundreds of thousands of men, women and children
around the world have been left to rot with wrong diagnoses,
or have had their Lyme disease acknowledged but been told that
it is an 'easily-treated' disease, given 3 weeks' antibiotics, then
told to shove off when their symptoms carried on after that.

In Britain the existence of the epidemic is denied complete-
ly, and virtually no effort made to warn or educate the public
about the dangers of ticks, which carry the bacteria Borrelia
burgdorferi.

The Borrelia genus has been a subject of bio war experimen-
tation at least as far back as WW2, when the infamous Japa-
nese Unit 731, which tortured and experimented on live pris-
oners, studied it.

The reality is, Lyme disease is for many a chronic, horren-
dous, incapacitating disease producing crippling fatigue, con-
stant pain, loss of memory, possible paralysis, psychosis, blind-
ness and even death.

It was an ideal bio war agent because it evades detection on
routine tests, has an enormous range of different presentations,

and can mimic everything from ADHD to multiple sclerosis to carpal tunnel syndrome to rheumatoid arthritis to chronic fatigue syndrome (M.E.) to lupus to schizophrenia. Enemy medical staff would never know what had hit them, nor even that ONE illness had hit their population, rather than an unexplained rise in dozens of known conditions.

Honest doctors and scientists who tried to treat or research Lyme disease according to ethical principles have been viciously persecuted by government-backed organizations in the US, Europe and elsewhere. Many specialists in the US were threatened with loss of their license or had anonymous, false allegations sent to the medical board, which tied them up in mountains of paperwork and legal fees... some were forced out of medicine or even driven to suicide.

Instead, medical disinfo agents, most of whom have a background in military/bio-warfare units, such as (names removed in this book, but you can see them online) etc. were enabled to assume top positions in Lyme research, CDC, NIH etc. from where they issued false information, covering up the true seriousness and chronic nature of the disease, and condemned untold numbers to a living hell.

Please help Lyme patients publicize this scandal, which has caused suffering on a massive scale. Contact me by email if you are interested in helping.

Thank you.
Lisa
E-mail: lymerayja@yahoo.co.uk

Welcome to the Club!

NOW YOU ARE ONE OF US, LABELED "INCURABLE"

ONLINE SUPPORT FORUMS

"*Without health life is not life; it is only a state of languor and suffering - an image of death.***"**

Buddha

From the first day I was diagnosed with Lyme, I was desperately searching for answers online. There are many forums and online communities that discuss treatments and protocols for Lyme. One of the biggest ones that I came across was *www.mdjunction.com*. I started reading all the posts and learning what treatments work and what don't. I have learned about Samento supplements from that forum and I have also learned that Lyme will make you miserable for the rest of your life. I had contacted "veterans" on that forum to ask them about what worked for them and the usual answer was that, *"Nothing worked and there was no cure."* It seems to me that people in the support groups are the ones who don't get better. Some of those people are cynical and depressed and they often tend to bring others down. I would often come across posts like: *"It is not worth it to even start treatments, because you will never get your health back anyways."* These skeptics are not a real representation of those of us who have actually healed from Lyme. While reading these posts, I was getting really depressed and discouraged however, I had that inner voice inside of me that knew there was some kind of solution and I would never give up.

I came across so many terrifying stories like: *"Cancer paled next to the despair of knowing I was facing this terrible dark place again – of constant pain, fatigue and whole body sickness. With cancer, I could still live life even though I might be facing death. But this illness was a living death."* Laurie Martin, a Californian who has struggled with both tick-borne infections and colon cancer, states that *"Cancer 'pales' in comparison to the pain and suffering of Lyme disease."*

So, I started searching for people with success stories ONLY and talking to those that healed themselves. Well, there were not many of them. (Most likely those who healed from Lyme simply moved on with their lives).I had found one lady on that forum. I remember her name was Connie. She was my hero, my inspiration, my hope. Connie was sick for at least 10 years before she got diagnosed, and she gave it all she had in an effort to heal herself! I was asking her questions every day about her treatments and supplements, and I was gaining a little hope to heal myself one day.

The most profound treatments for her were hydrogen peroxide IVs, vitamin C IVs, herbal detox supplements, and most importantly a radical life style change! She followed a strict raw-vegan diet, exercised, and practiced yoga as much as she could.

Connie was one out of thousands of members on *www. mdjunction.com* who had a success story, and she was very positive and helpful. Everybody else seemed depressed and hopeless. They were very negative and had a nasty attitude. They were complaining about the usual stuff: insurance does not pay, doctors do not know anything, and life sucks! All of them were VICTIMS and only Connie was a WARRIOR! I had decided I was not going to join a "victim" community and that I would be a warrior, too!

While experimenting with different treatments and protocols, I would go back to *www.mdjunction.com* and post an inspiring message about a treatment or protocol that worked for me. Apparently, it would get deleted in a few hours by a "group manager" and my account would get blocked. First I thought that it was some kind of Internet malfunction. I created a new user name and posted the same message again – and guess what, it got deleted right away and my account got blocked again! Apparently, the "group manager" decides what posts to approve and what not to. So I asked her why my posts were getting deleted. Her answer was basically that Lyme is incurable; she had been on that forum for years and no one ever reported any improvement from that particular treatment or herb I was talking about, and I am not supposed to post any product name because it looks like I am endorsing that specific product. She accused me of being a charlatan, trying to make money off of poor people by advertising a certain product or treatment. So how are we supposed to help other people and talk about what treatments worked for us?

There are also some great forums out there, my favorite is *www.curezone.com*. To this day I refer to *Curezone* to research different treatments, supplements, and cleanses and to read inspirational stories.

The moral of the story is – find people with success stories that you can learn from and copy what they have done to heal themselves. Do not get discouraged by the forums and "victims" that complain all day long about how unfortunate they are. As you can see, it is hard to find any reliable information on what products work and which do not on *mdjunction.com*, because forum policy does not allow contributors to name the product. And members of that forum are very negative. They are not willing to change their attitude and they are comfortable just playing "victim" for several reasons: they would not have to take any responsibility for their own health, they get to stay home all day long while their spouses are taking care of them, they can complain and people feel sorry for them, etc. I encourage all of you, my friends, to avoid falling prey to a "victim" mentality and instead look for the gifts in your healing journey!

I had found four people online, (by the way all of them are women) who I was learning from. Those women were tough; they were warriors and I learned how to become a warrior and stay a warrior even during the worst flare-ups.

Taking Full Responsibility for Your Health

66There are NO incurable diseases, NONE. Take **RESPONSIBILITY**, *and be willing to* **CHANGE**, *and you can heal yourself of anything.* 99

Dr. Schulze

So before we move any further, this chapter is an absolute MUST!

When I first became sick I was constantly crying and asking: *"Why me?"* And I was desperately looking for a "cure". I was researching treatments and protocols hoping there would be some special treatment like stem cell therapy, for instance, that would cure me.

Sound familiar?

Most of us are asking the wrong questions and playing "victims". You cannot get better if you do not change your attitude! I do not care how many antibiotics you are going to take and what fancy treatments you are undergoing, you simply won't get better if you do not take full responsibility of your health and change your attitude!

No more asking: "Why me?" Who even cares? All you need right now is to get better! From now on you will ask yourself: What can I do TODAY to improve my health? How can I support my immune system? What treatments are more aligned with me – conventional or alternative, or both? How can I support my mind? What am I grateful for?

Every time you feel discouraged, repeat this affirmation: *"My body is able to heal itself. My body is designed to heal itself. Nothing is incurable!"*

When I was sick I printed out the following two quotes that always reminded me I was going to get well no matter what!

"I believe the body can heal itself if given the proper stimulus! Lyme disease is no exception! It makes sense to try an approach that will work WITH your immune system instead of against it. Never settle for being told that something is incurable! Get Empowered! Get Well!" Dr. Cindee Gardner

And the second one was: *"When you want something, all the universe conspires in helping you to achieve it."* P. Coelho

You can use my quotes or find your own that will inspire you and remind you that you WILL get better no matter what!

"I have consistently seen that people who are able to get rid of their anger heal. Those who are eaten up with anger and resentment, as well those who get depressed and ask questions like, 'Why me?' don't tend to heal." Dr. Ginger Savely, DNP

I was desperately looking for a cure. I was researching treatments and protocols hoping there would be some special treatment like Multi Wave Oscillator or some other fancy device that would cure me. The whole business of medicine brainwashed us in to the idea of "finding" a cure. The word "finding" implies to look outside yourself for the answer. We were taught that healing is a matter of finding the right cure for your particular disease. Lately it has become more obvious that health is a personal responsibility. Medicine has become a lucrative business, guided by the pharmaceutical companies. They've managed to put people in a constant state of fear; always worrying about the next disease or epidemic.

I suggest taking back responsibility and authority for yourself. Educating yourself about health and how the body functions can be very empowering.

I have to disappoint you my friends -- There is NO magic pill.

You, not your doctor (healer, herbalist, shaman, etc.) YOU are going to need to take full responsibility for your own health! No one is as interested in getting you well as yourself.

A doctor can prescribe you treatments, antibiotics, herbs, however you need to step up and do all the heavy lifting! The lifestyle changes I will list in this book are an absolute MUST if you want to regain your health back and kiss your "Lyme" good-bye.

Remember, we are all unique and some treatments that worked for me might not work for you and vice versa, however you will never know unless you give each of them a good try. All life style changes are absolutely necessary in order to heal yourself.

Are you ready? Are you ready to take responsibility and dive into a healing journey? And I don't promise it is going to be easy. As a matter of fact, it is NOT going to be easy! It is going to be hard work with moments of disappointment and feelings of giving up. During those moments you need to stay strong, because you are a warrior and YOU WILL WIN THIS BATTLE - WHATEVER IT TAKES!

Medical Prognosis

❝Doctors give drugs of which they know little, into bodies, of which they know less, for diseases of which they know nothing at all. ❞

Voltaire

No matter what prognosis your MD gave you – YOU can REVERSE MOST MEDICAL CONDITIONS! Medical prognoses are based on the outcome of the AVERAGE person who has this particular disease.

YOU are NOT an AVERAGE person!

You might still doubt there is a possibility to get well because your doctor (or even dozens of them) gave you some kind of medical prognosis and told you there was little chance of recovering from chronic Lyme and you'll be lucky if it ever goes into remission. I know; I've been there.

I was told by so many doctors that I had little to no chance of recovering from chronic Lyme. And you know what; those statistics and medical prognoses are based on an AVERAGE person. They could be true, but again, medical prognoses are based on the outcome of the AVERAGE person who has this particular disease. And YOU are NOT an AVERAGE person!

Let's see who an AVERAGE person is.

In one year, an AVERAGE person:

- Eats low-nutrition, high fat and sugar, over processed, nutritionally depleted = junk food.
- Consumes 300 soft drinks
- 170 pounds of white sugar
- 400 candy bars
- 500 donuts

In an AVERAGE person's lifetime they consume:

- 12 entire 3,000 pound cows
- 6 whole pigs
- 3,000 chickens
- 3,000 fish/seafood
- 30,000 quarts of milk

They also:

- Average 2-4 bowel movements a week (70,000 bowel movements in a lifetime!)
- Experience none or very little exercise
- Are 25 pounds or more overweight
- Suffer from high blood pressure
- Consume over 30,000 aspirin and other painkillers in a lifetime
- Consume over 20,000 OTC & prescription medications
- Drink over 2,000 gallons of alcohol
- Have a negative self-image
- Experience bouts of anxiety/depression

The AVERAGE American is physically, emotionally, and spiritually sick.

Therefore, the doctor's prognosis could be somewhat correct.

However, you are NOT an AVERAGE person! You have decided to change and take full responsibility for your health, right? In his book called, *Creating Health*, Deepak Chopra, MD states the following, "*I have frequently observed that a rapid progression of symptoms and then death from cancer occurred after the diagnosis of cancer was made. It is almost as if the patient was dying from the diagnosis and not from the disease.*" This is sad, especially when we just learned that medical diagnoses tend to be WRONG! Moreover, often physicians psychologically damage their patients. When doctors estimate how long a patient will live, or predict that the patient will never walk or see again, they can create a self-fulfilling prophecy.

"*The word incurable is modern. I suspect coined by allopaths. The word incurable is not found in any indigenous language. Translated it means: I do not know how to cure you. But instead of taking the responsibility to tell you that, or refer you to someone who might be able to help with your cure, I will instead guilt trip you and blame YOU for being incurable and ruining my day.* "D.

Absolute Faith

66Every tomorrow has two handles. We can take hold of it with the handle of anxiety or the handle of faith. 99

Henry Ward Beecher

This brings us to another very important topic - FAITH.

No matter how sick you get while 'herxing'*, no matter how bad your flare-ups are, you must always have an Absolute Faith that you are getting better! You always know your body is able to heal itself if given the PROPER STIMULUS. You will take an approach that will work WITH YOUR IMMUNE SYSTEM, instead of against it.

"The person that fully heals is the one who has the right attitude and support system, and who doesn't believe he or she will always be ill. If people believe that there is a chance they will eventually be well, then it is more likely that they will. A lot of patients have been told by well-intentioned practitioners that they will always be sick, and so if they believe what the practitioner says, then they won't get well."
Dr. Lee Cowden, MD

As I mentioned in an earlier chapter, every time I was feeling discouraged, I would read success stories of those who reversed their degenerative diseases. And not just Lyme, but cancer, AIDS, MS, chronic digestion problems, allergies, you name it. I would repeat positive affirmations that my body is able to heal itself, and I would also find as many things and moments in my life to be grateful for as possible.

All of those methods are wonderful methods in conditioning our mind and creating a positive environment for our bodies to heal. By the way, the most acidic thing for our body is not even meat, coffee or alcohol; it is hatred, and the most alkalizing is not a wheatgrass shot, but gratitude and love! So I was already practicing all of the above positive methods, and I was feeling pretty good. I was slowly recovering but I felt like I hit a plateau. I had days when I was really skeptical if I would ever recover completely.

But something happened that changed my belief system forever. I bought tickets to Tony Robbins seminar, "Unleash the Power Within." I remember every detail of that event as if it just happened yesterday. First of all, I was BEYOND impressed with this man called Tony Robbins. If you do not know him, Mr. Robbins healed himself of a brain tumor with major lifestyle changes. (Just one more success story that I researched and applied to myself) Tony Robbins is a huge guy; about 6 ft. 7 inches tall and very muscular. And no, he does not take any artificial protein supplements nor does he eat meat. Mr. Tony Robbins does not eat any animal products, basically he is a vegan. What really blew my mind was that Tony Robbins was on stage for 15 hours each day for four days in a row. During the 15-hour day, Mr. Robbins did not sit down once. He did not drink, eat, or leave to use a bathroom. And on top of that, he had an unstoppable energy! I realized if this pure unstoppable energy is possible for one human being, it is possible for any of us! I made it my life goal to create such a lifestyle that generates optimum health and unlimited pure energy for others and for me. To this day Mr. Tony Robbins is my role model.

However the unlimited energy and vibrant health of Mr. Robbins was not the only thing that blew my mind. By the end of day one, we were conditioned and trained that ANYTHING IS POSSIBLE and our BODY IS CAPABLE OF ANYTHING. You might think: What is she talking about? Well, after the first 15-hour day, 3,000 of us went outside to perform the famous "fire walk". To tell you I was scared is an understatement. I was TERRIFIED! We were standing in line in front of a row of burning coals. And one by one we were walking on them. Just to compare, your cooking stove is about 600 degrees Fahrenheit's, the burning coals are over 2, 000 (!) degrees Fahrenheit! Now this seems impossible, right? I was about to run away but I told myself: *"If I can walk on burning coals without hurting myself – I will experience the truth that my body is capable of anything, which means I will be able to recover from Lyme for good! The worst case is that I'll burn my feet, but what are burned feet compared to living with Lyme??"*

There are no words to describe my feelings on the other end of the fire walk. I was jumping up and down, screaming, and hugging people. At that moment I knew — NOTHING IS IMPOSSIBLE! Something had shifted in my brain and I was 100% confident I would beat Lyme and it was just a matter of time. And in order to speed up healing I became 100% committed to implementing all lifestyle changes that would create my optimum health. Faith had rooted itself in my heart and mind in my body's ability to recover.

"*Step into a New World. A world without chronic diseases. Step out of your old world. It has kept you a prisoner. Try something new! The prison has no walls. It has only lines that mark the ground around you. Inside the lines are your old ideas. Dare to step out and try new ideas and your illness promises to recede. In a few weeks it can be gone.*" Hulda Clark

According to the Merriam-Webster definition, a Herxheimer reaction is caused as a direct result of using spirocheticidal drugs (mainly antibiotics) to treat individuals with a spirochetal disease which results in an increase in the symptoms of the treated condition. Dorlands Medical Dictionary adds that the condition is a short term immunological reaction which causes fever, chills, muscle pain, headaches, and skin lesions. Both Adolph Jerisch, an Australian dermatologist, and Karl Herxheimer, a German dermatologist, are credited with the discovery of the condition, although Jerisch published his findings in1895, seven years earlier than his brother.

Let's get straight to business...

GET RID OF YOUR STORY FIRST AND FOR GOOD.

> **"**It is in your moments of decision that your destiny is shaped....**"**
>
> Tony Robbins

I have tried everything – nothing works! There is no cure, why even bother? Maybe next year they will come up with a "magic" pill. I have no energy to exercise. I have no money to buy organic food.

So which one are you? Which one is your story? Because you know – your story is just a story that can be changed in a heartbeat. It is your mindset, your belief system and your excuse. And all of the above comes from fear. The number one obstacle that stops people from getting what they want is fear. Fear to fail (you are afraid the next treatment will fail you), fear of pain (you are afraid you'll get worse before you get better), fear of the unknown (you are afraid of the outcomes of the next protocol). You can tell yourself a story that you don't have energy, money, resources, but in reality you are afraid.

I have a friend that I met online from New York. It had been a year since I was diagnosed and I was still a mess; but I was better compared to how I started. We had been talking for about seven months on the phone almost every single day before we finally met. I was getting better and better and his condition was not changing. I asked him, *"So, what treatments are you doing, what protocols are you taking to get better?"* He said, *"Nothing, I have tried it all. I have been sick for many years, nothing works. I need strong drugs to cure me, I do not believe in all those woo-woo treatments."* So I asked him, *"Have you tried Ozone and it did not work for you?"* *"No, I have not tried that,"* he replied. *"Have you tried a Rife machine?"* I asked. *"No, I have not."* *"Have you tried ACT?"* – *"No, but I do not believe in that program, it is not scientifically explainable,"* he insisted. As you can see, this person said he already tried everything and nothing works, apparently he tried one or two treatments and gave up. Also, he had been sick for six years and doing nothing to recover. So how does he expect to get better?

A few months later I started bugging him to try modified Gerson therapy. His reply was, *"I can't. I have no time. I cannot juice fast, I will be hungry and I have no time for coffee enemas."* But you know me by now, I never give up. I called him once and offered another option. I said, *"How about you come to San Diego and stay with me. I will be juicing for you and you can just stay, relax, and go to the beach. It is a very healing environment in Southern California; I know it will help you."* What do you think his response was? That's right, *"I can't. I have too many responsibilities, I have bills to pay, and I have to help out my mother."* This person is full of excuses and he is not willing to get out of his comfort zone (which is extremely uncomfortable by the way! I don't think it's comfortable to live with chronic pains, fatigue and exhaustion).

Well, it did not stop me from trying to help him. I decided to convince him to go 100% raw vegan to boost his immune system if he *"can't"* juice fast. Of course he came up with an excuse right away, *"It is too cold in New York for raw foods. There are no places to eat raw by where I live. I want to be 'normal', I want to eat and drink what everybody else is eating and drinking."*

Then a few months later I went to a detox and cleanse retreat. It was really affordable to anyone and extremely powerful. In a week of detox I felt like I took a giant step forward towards my optimum health (this is how I created the program for our *Health Mastery Retreats*, because the results I got were incredible!)

On my way home I called him since I was super excited to tell him about this program that could totally transform his life. You know his answer. Of course he never gave it a shot.

And there are tons of people like that. I would say the majority of people that contact me are not willing to change!

So, it's been two years since him and I met. Here I am—healthy, happy, running my own business, launching a new business, writing this book, and him – still sick and tired, barely putting up with his same job. This is your choice, my friends. You decide if you want to be a warrior or a victim.

From my inbox:

Good morning Katrina,

My name is Susie and I am ridding myself of this thing called Lyme.

I'm doing fantastic!

I've treated ALL naturally through intense treatments in Reno and through DIET, ATTITUDE, and mostly, God!

It is not a quick fix, as you may know!

Could you call me at your earliest convenience?

Thank you so much, and thrilled to hear you are symptom free!!!

Suzie

❧ ❧

Re: Lyme disease Victim

"So I am fairly sure I am a Lyme victim...and I am trying to write down a list of my symptoms...

My joints are really hurting me in the wrist and elbows but they don't have redness all the time I have only noticed a little redness in my thumb joints and none in my elbows...

Is this common?... I would like my doctor to see that I have joint pain...but I hear usually it comes with swelling and redness most of the time...

Behind my knees hurt off and on...I do plan on seeing a LLMD as soon as I can get enough money...which could take a while...ugh."

Anonymous

You can clearly see two different attitudes of two young women that are dealing with Lyme. The first one, Suzie, will recover pretty soon, her positive attitude will help!

The second one will have a challenging time till she changes her state from a "victim" to a "warrior".

There are 3 main steps to get results (whether it is your health, your finances, your body, your relationship or your business).

1. You need a new strategy.

If you are sick and not getting better – you need a new strategy.

2. You need a better story.

If you are sick and your story is, *"I have no energy, I have no finances, and there is no cure,"* you need to come up with a better story like, *"I am going to start a new treatment. I know there is no 'overnight cure', but day by day I am getting better and better. I know that my body can heal itself, and I will do whatever it takes to assist it."* This is your new story!

3. You need a better state (in your body, mind, and emotions).

I know that we have bad days and VERY bad days. I've been there. No matter how tired I was and how much my body ached, I would make myself exercise. If I could not jog, I would go for a walk. If I could not do yoga, I would do a gentle stretch at home. If I got depressed, I would look at my affirmations on the wall and repeat them as many times as necessary to change my emotional state. If I got discouraged, I would reread successful stories over and over again and tell myself than I am getting my health back - whatever it takes!

You have two choices, my friends; you can **choose** to stay the way you are right now – sick and tired, or you can **choose** to take charge of your life and apply the steps I am giving you in this book. This is your life, and this is your choice. You either choose to take full responsibility for your own health or you choose to be a victim.

And I am here to help. In order to succeed in any area of your life (health, business, relationship), you need a role model to know that what you are striving for is real and attainable. You need to find someone who has already achieved the results you are aiming for and model his/her behavior. In my case, I found four warriors who healed themselves from chronic Lyme the natural way without pharmaceutical drugs, and I followed their pattern. And you have to be "hungry" enough to do that, too. In life you need either an inspiration or desperation and I had them both. I encourage you to apply all steps I will give you in Part 2 of this book to assist you on your way to optimum health.

The moment you decide that you are 100% committed to getting your health back, no obstacle, no challenge, and no problem will keep you from it. In that moment your life will change forever, and you will be empowered to take control!

"If you believe you can or if you believe you can't, you are right." Henry Ford

And now it's time to discuss the "PROPER STIMULI" and approaches that will work **WITH** YOUR IMMUNE SYSTEM.

A Look at Supplements

ANTIBIOTICS – CURE OR POISON?

❝What is impossible to see from the viewpoint of those who believe in cures is that the very symptoms the good doctors have suppressed and turned into chronic disease were the body's only means of correcting the problem! The so-called 'disease' was the only 'cure' possible! ❞

Dr. Philip Chapman

I started Doxycycline the same day I was diagnosed by the neurologist. I do not believe in drugs and never take any. However, this time I have decided to step over my beliefs; choosing the lesser evil. What I was going through was a zillion times worse than the side effects of antibiotics. I have to note however, it is very important that a treatment is aligned with you. If you do believe in pharmaceutical drugs like antibiotics, they might actually work for you.

As you may have guessed, 90 days of Doxycycline did not do me any good; otherwise this book would be complete right here. Unfortunately, I was getting worse and worse during those three months. My LLMD told me to start another three antibiotics plus Mepron for Babesia for another five months! I knew I did not want to experiment with drugs anymore so I stopped seeing my LLMD and took my healing in to my own hands.

I had decided not to take any more antibiotics for the following reasons:

First off, antibiotic means, "against life" which does not align with my vision of healing - at all.

Those four women that healed themselves reported that antibiotics had failed them, and moreover they even felt much worse afterwards.

Since Lyme spirochetes can become cysts virtually instantaneously in the presence of threatening antibiotics, it does not make sense to use antibiotics.

Antibiotics are too large and are not able to cross the blood-brain barrier, and most of my symptoms were affecting my brain.

Antibiotics are not able to get into joints, bones, and other tissue, where spirochete hides.

And last, but not least, antibiotics suppress the immune system - big time.

In order to promote the body's ability to heal, Lyme warriors must do everything possible to strengthen their immune system.

Remember, it makes sense to take an approach that will work WITH YOUR IMMUNE SYSTEM, instead of against it. And antibiotics were working AGAINST my immune system.

"I consider the use of antibiotic medications for the treatment of Lyme disease and other infections to be highly ques-

tionable. People with Lyme frequently observe positive changes in their symptoms as a result of antibiotic use, yet they are only that: a shift in symptoms. They may still have bacteria in their cells. But these may not be reflected in their lab results or symptoms – they may only be detected by some type of energetic testing. Most patients who have gone into remission from Lyme disease after antibiotic use have later suffered from other diseases, due to the immune suppression that the medications cause. Such diseases are seemingly unrelated to Lyme but were probably initially caused by Lyme. I have observed, for instance, that there is an increase in patients' risk of developing cancer after they have been on long-term antibiotics.

In any case, I believe that antibiotics prevent or hinder the defense system of the cell, and I haven't observed any cases of complete healing from Lyme disease as a result of antibiotic therapy." Dr. Ingo D.E. Woitzel, MD

"Another problem with antibiotics is that they don't deal with the core problem, which is a weak immune system and consequent susceptibility to illness. Antibiotics are toxic to many organs of the body and can damage the kidneys, ears, gastrointestinal tract, and liver. Their use comes at a high cost." Ronald Whitmont, MD

So this was my decision to heal myself without the use of any pharmaceutical drugs. From day one I knew antibiotics were not aligned with me. This is your personal choice. Please use common sense, research, and interview people; ask your body what it needs. Your belief system must be in sync with your treatment plan. Otherwise, cognitive dissonance might prevent your body from accessing its own healing mechanism.

I do believe in applied kinesiology - muscle testing. Hey, even in Dr. Raxlen's office I was diagnosed with Lyme on my first visit by a muscle test, even though he is a western medical doc and prescribes drugs.

Cowden Protocol

"Most diseases are the result of medication which has been prescribed to relieve and take away a beneficent and warning symptom on the part of Nature. "

Elbert Hubbard

While I was on Doxycycline, I added modified Cowden protocol. I was taking most of the herbs from the protocol, but not all. Dr. Cowden's protocols for treating Lyme disease can be found at: *www.bionatus.com/nutramedix.*

For me that was not an "overnight" cure, but I did feel subtle improvements. I did, however, experience fantastic results with the use of Samento, when I was coming down with a cold. Usually I would at least sneeze a few days and get a runny nose. Not anymore. When I would feel the first sign of a cold coming on, I would take Samento and all the common cold symptoms would disappear within a few hours. The herbs in the Cowden protocol are very potent and unlike pharmaceutical drugs, herbs work on many levels at the same time. Any herb has more than just one function. For example, Samento is an herbal antibiotic so it kills bugs and at the same time Samento is a phenomenal immune system booster. Samento has shown dramatic benefits in virtually every kind of inflammation. It reverses most asthma and arthritis cases and helps the body fight acute infections from AIDS to Hepatitis, and has even been found to help manage most forms of cancer.

Unlike antibiotics, the human body does not develop a resistance to herbal antibiotics. However, you do need to switch protocols after 4-8 months to target different bugs. *"Relapses are less common with herbal therapy if patients are treated appropriately and for the right length of time, based on energetic evaluation,"* Dr. Lee Cowden, MD

I do recommend the Cowden protocol. As I have stated in the previous chapter, we are all unique. And what does not work for one person might work for you. I have read many success stories with Samento and I believe that this is one of the herbs you should give a chance to.

"Dr. James Schaller, MD, MAR (LLMD) found that there was no pharmaceutical drug that worked consistently to eliminate all species of Bartonella in these patients, and that only three types of herbal remedies could do the job. Those remedies were Cumanda, clove bud oil, and Houttuynia herb from China."

I have met so many people that quit too early. They complain that nothing works. I really encourage you to stick to a treatment or to a protocol for at least two months or even longer before you decide it does not work for you. Lyme is a tricky disease. Most people feel worse when first starting a certain protocol and because of this, they think that it is not working so they quit and jump to another treatment. You see, most likely they are experiencing Herxheimer's reaction, meaning that the treatment is indeed working by killing lots of bugs – this is a good thing! Be patient.

Artemisinin for Babesia

"Ignorance and arrogance make a bad combination, and 'modern' medicine has been guilty of both for decades. The news media have been their willing accomplices. The misinformation they spew to this day is fraught with fabricated frights of natural therapies, while in the same breath they spew forth the wonders of pharmaceutical drugs."

Andrew Saul

While my Western Blot came up negative for Babesiosis, I was diagnosed with a co-infection by clinical manifestations. I had severe night sweats that were so bad that I had to get up twice a night to change my shirt because it was soaking wet. Also, my pillow and my blanket were wet. I experienced the misery of alternating between chills and hot flashes, plus shortness of breath.

I was prescribed Mepron for Babesiosis, and my LLMD also mentioned the herb called Artemisinin. Since I was already on Doxycycline for 40 days and I was not improving one bit, I decided not to add any more pharmaceutical drugs and I went the natural route. I was taking Artemisinin for six weeks straight. After about four weeks my night sweats stopped and two weeks later I decided to stop Artemisinin. It was one of the most potent herbs so far on my way to healing. Also I have to note, I was prescribed triple the amount of the manufacturer's suggested dose. Consult your practitioner for your dosage.

Date at the IV Room, Nutritional IVs

While my night sweats were gone, my other symptoms were getting worse. By that time I did not really know if I was getting worse or if I was 'herxing'. So I continued researching doctors hoping someone had some "hidden" treatment that would cure me. I found another LLMD at a pretty busy clinic on 42Nd Street in Manhattan. That clinic looked very different from other medical offices that were also treating Lyme. The clinic looked very fancy, like a high-end spa, which was really emotionally uplifting for me; unlike previous small, old, and depressing offices. And my first visit did not cost that much compared to other doctors; I paid $470 for this particular visit.

The doctor I was there to see was very knowledgeable in western medicine, as well as alternative medicine. He took his time asking many questions and learning a lot about me. After the intake part, we moved into the treatment room. He performed a good amount of muscle testing on me; covering different diseases, all my internal organs and their functioning and testing my beliefs on different treatments. Apparently, my body was very weak to antibiotics and I was kind of relieved to learn that because I was planning to go the natural route after my course of Doxycycline. After the muscle testing I underwent oxygen chamber therapy. The session lasted about an hour and I was feeling pretty uncomfortable being in a closed capsule. I truly believe oxygen (Hyperbaric Oxygen Therapy) is very powerful and has tremendous healing properties. However it was pricey, as well. I was not able to afford continued oxygen treatments since I already had a tremendous amount of expenses for supplements, other treatments and doctor visits. After the oxygen therapy I was sent to the IV room. That was quite an experience! I have seen many IV rooms before that, but this one stands out! It did look like an upscale spa and the chair I was sitting in was like the pedicure massage chairs with all kinds of massage options. You could not find any medical reading material; instead they had *Cosmopolitan*, *People*, *Shape*, and other popular magazines for women and *Wall Street Journal*, *New York Times*, and other newspapers for finance folks. Even the patients were different! No one looked like a terminal AIDS or cancer patient. Everyone looked pretty good and what amazed me was that everyone was working on their laptops and 'smartphones'. That's amazing – even Lyme (or some other chronic illness) does not stop a New Yorker from their busy life! And another guy sitting next to me with his IV (young and good looking by the way) was trying to pick me up, right there, in the IV room. Before I used to get my dates at fashion shows or fitness and nutrition events, and now I was being asked on a date at a doctor's office that treats HIV, AIDS, CFS, Lyme, and other scary disorders… what an experience!

In this same medical office I was prescribed "RN Transfer Factor Lyme plus" and homeopathic Lyme nosode, as well Buhner's herbal protocol. (A nosode is a homeopathic remedy prepared from a pathological specimen. A nosode will create an informatory/energetic protection from the microbes. Nosodes can also help to recover old and almost 'forgotten' infectious diseases, which never have been cured completely). I was taking those two medicines for almost three months before I stopped. The reason I stopped "RN Transfer Factor Lyme plus" was because it was pretty expensive and I thought I could invest that money on more potent medicine. (Again, more potent for me. Remember, if it did not work for me it does not mean it won't work for you!) And I stopped homeopathic nosode because I had decided to find a homeopath that practices "Classical" homeopathy and get a prescription based on my body constitution and on my clinical manifestation.

I would like to mention that nutritional IVs, especially vitamin C are very powerful. I had only experienced a few of them, but I have interviewed other patients in IV rooms and they all confirmed IVs were making a huge difference for them. Also some people took hydrogen peroxide IVs and they swear by them. I have not tried them since I was doing so many other treatments; I did not want to overload. Also, I had decided to put all kinds of IVs aside and only consider using them as emergency treatments if nothing else worked since they were a little too invasive for me.

Buhner's Protocol

I was told to follow Buhner's protocol by two LLMDs and multiple Naturopaths. Since I was an Oriental Medicine student at that time, I was already familiar with the herbs and their functions, so I could tell his protocol was pretty powerful.

The core protocol consists of Andrographis paniculata, Cat's Claw, and Japanese Knotweed. Optional "core" additions are Astragalus and Sarsaparilla. I'll talk about these in a bit, but you really need to read his book *Healing Lyme*.

ANDROGRAPHIS

- Anti-spirochetal (Brain: calming agent)
- Immune booster and modulator
- Anti-inflammatory
- Enhances cognitive function
- Lessens fatigue
- Enhances liver function
- Anti-inflammatory for arthritis symptoms
- Enhances liver function, helping to clear infection from the body
- Reduces Lyme endotoxin damage

- Easily crosses blood/brain barrier and specifically protects brain from inflammatory damage and Lyme toxins

CAT'S CLAW

- Immune booster
- Anti-inflammatory - arthritis and muscle pain
- Enhances central nervous system and cognitive function
- Increases CD57 white blood cell count (natural killer cells)
-

POLYGONUM (KNOTWEED, HU ZHANG) SMILAX (SARSAPARILLA)

- Binds toxins, helping to flush them and reduce Herx symptoms
- Eleuthero (Siberian Ginseng)
- Immune system booster
- Adrenal tonic
- Antidepressant, mental clarity stimulant
- Enhances energy levels
- Adaptogen: increases nonspecific resistance to adverse influences

Mr. Buhner recommends relatively high doses of these herbs. Without the book, and just a list of herbs, or from talking to someone in a health food store, I would never have guessed to take so much. To temper this, as I believe there may be some digestive upset at first, he suggests increasing the dose gradually over four to five weeks. Then, at full strength, continuing for *at least* two months, and more likely 8-12 months, depending on symptoms. Eventually reverse the process, slowly stepping down the dosage, to either none or to a maintenance level.

As I stated earlier in the chapter, Artemisinin (derived from Artemesia) is one of the most powerful herbs. I was able to get rid of the Babesiosis infection within two months. Andrographis was one of the main herbs for me as well. It is such a potent herb and it not only kills the bugs, but also enhances the immune system. And instead of Cat's Claw I was taking Samento, which is TOA (tetracyclic oxindole alkaloids) – free Cat's Claw.

I truly believe Buhner's protocol played a significant role in my recovery.

Ondamed: The Wonder Device

Thanks to Carolyn, the PA at Dr. Raxlen's office, I had learned about Ondamed right away; which is an electromagnetic pulsed biofeedback therapy device. What a powerful machine! Ondamed is like a Rife machine but more advanced. It has a biofeedback device installed so it finds what your body needs and what frequencies to use. It uses electromagnetic frequencies to balance the body and kill the bugs.

I have found about 12 Ondamed practitioners in NYC. Some of them would charge $300 per session, so I would not even consider them. The rest charged $120 and up. First I went to the practitioner that lived closest to me on the Lower East Side. It turned out to be an older Jewish couple that had all kinds of equipment at home. They were very friendly and also took their time to learn about me (or they were just bored and my story was quite entertaining for them). Finally they escorted me to their guestroom where the "Ondamed" machine was. The wife proceeded to read the instructions to her husband on how to use the device as the husband tried to get it to work. Also, they were asking weird and unrelated questions. As the man was scanning my body, all of a sudden he said, "Yes, you were right… you do not have hemorrhoids." In that moment I was done with those practitioners!

The next day I went to see another healer with an "On-damed" machine. She was really great and I continued to feel the difference with each treatment. Again, it was not an overnight cure; however at least I was feeling better during and after the treatment. This particular woman (her name was Lainey) was super knowledgeable in all kinds of natural healing modalities and she introduced me to a lot of interesting information that I did not know before. For example, I learned about "Two Feathers Healing Formula", Oil Pulling Therapy, MMS and other great modalities.

As a bonus, during each "Ondamed" treatment, Lainey performed on me both Craniosacral therapy and sound healing with Tibetan bowls. I just loved my sessions with her. I felt healing energy in her environment.

I completed three sessions per week for six months in a row of the Ondamed treatments before I moved to San Diego. I know for sure Ondamed treatments have helped me a lot by killing the bugs as well as enhancing my overall immune system.

Acupuncture

Directly following my Ondamed treatments I usually had an acupuncture treatment by a practitioner who was basically next door to Lainey's house. I loved my acupuncture sessions. The practitioner was phenomenal (she was one of my professors at my acupuncture school at the time). Her name was Anne Jeffres, and if she ever reads this book and remembers me, I would like to let her know how grateful I am for her treatments!

I highly recommend getting regular acupuncture treatments. Lyme is so harsh on our bodies that we get out of balance easily. Acupuncture helps bring the body into balance, as well as provides numerous other benefits.

Oriental medicine is a holistic approach, which is based on the treatment of all bodily systems. Acupuncture benefits the improvement of physical health conditions and is affective on many disorders. It also instills a feeling of increased mental clarity.

Acupuncture works directly with the body's energy or qi (chi), as acupuncture practitioners believe that all illnesses are a result of the natural flow of energy through the body becoming stuck, depleted or weakened and thus making the individual susceptible to illness. Acupuncture benefits the rebalance of qi through the treatment of specific acupoints related to symptoms or illnesses that are present. Acupuncture treatments are effective in removing these energy obstructions.

With certain health conditions, acupuncture can be effective enough to reduce or eliminate the need to take drugs to control pain or symptoms. Additional benefits of acupuncture include: faster recovery from injuries, decreased symptoms of stress and improved circulation.

Acupuncture treatment benefits the immune system by strengthening the overall functioning of it. By utilizing this type of treatment it means that the immune system is better able to withstand colds, infections, and the flu.

Dr. Zhang and Modern Chinese Medicine

Again, I would like to thank Carolyn Welcome from Dr. Raxlen's office for referring me to Dr. Zhang. I called his office right away to schedule an appointment; however he was booked out two months in advance. His receptionist on the phone was very nice. She told me to go online to his website and order his herbs under "Lyme protocol".

I did order the herbs from Dr. Zhang's protocol. You can find more information about his protocol at *www.sinomedresearch.org.* Dr. Zhang's formulas are very potent and of great quality (somewhat pricey though). I added his protocol on top of Dr. Cowden's protocol.

When the time arrived, I went to see Dr. Zhang in his Manhattan office. And please, don't get me wrong here – I really respect Dr. Zhang and I think he is one of the most knowledgeable doctors in Oriental Medicine. However, my experience was a little weird. When I came in, he showed me an article from some old newspaper on the benefits of acupuncture. He was trying to persuade me that some studies show that acupuncture has many benefits. He also showed me pictures of the human brain before and after the treatment. First of all, if I did not believe in acupuncture I would not be sitting in his office. And secondly, I repeated to him several times that I was an acupuncture student myself and to say that 'I believe in acupuncture' is an understatement. Then he told me to use his herbal protocol that I had already been using and he escorted me to the treatment room where his assistant was needling me.

Again, I would like to state that Dr. Zhang is not only very knowledgeable in Oriental Medicine he is considered one of the best. Although my experience in his office did not feel like a healing experience – it was kind of rushed and impersonal. I would recommend finding an acupuncturist that has a healing ambience in his/her clinic and who will spend as much time with you as you need.

Two Feathers Healing Formula

As I had mentioned in the *Ondamed* chapter, I learned about *Two Feathers Healing Formula* from my healer Lainey. She described this medicine as something super powerful. Lainey also warned me that when I ingest it, most likely I will become very sick and it will feel like, *"I am dying."*

Oh well, I was feeling like I was dying anyway, so I had nothing to lose. I shut down the lights, burned some candles and incense, put on meditation music, and only took a small dose of "Two Feathers". As I'm lying there waiting to become immediately sick, I soon began to feel very sleepy (I am not sure if it was usual Lyme fatigue or if it was due to the high mineral content in the remedy) and I fell asleep. The next morning I woke without any abnormal sensation from the medicine.

Two Feathers Healing Formula is an American Indian healing formula that is over one hundred years old. It has been used to effectively treat allergies, diabetes, cancer, tumors, herpes, Chronic Fatigue Syndrome, liver detoxification, lupus, moles, parasites, skin cancers, vaginitis, viral diseases, yeast & fungal infections, and worms. It can also be used as a potent preventative remedy and detoxifier.

"Two Feathers Healing Formula is a unique formula that has reached through time, over several hundred years, to meet the needs of an ailing civilization today. It is like a time capsule sent to us from a distant past when knowledge was more of the spirit than of the intellect. There is a great sincerity and respect for this healing formula at every stage of its preparation. Those who handle the compound, including myself, feel blessed to be a part of an age-old rite that is indeed very special. Still produced in the original Native American manner, each herb is cured in smoke ovens and mixed in wooden bowls. Metal is never allowed to touch the formula as it would destabilize the electrolysis process provided by the components in the compound." Robert Roy

I have spoken with Robert Roy, the man who makes this medicine. Robert is a very wise and humble man. He is all about a healthy lifestyle and he is happy to help. I remember calling him and telling him that I'd been on the formula for the past four months and I still had symptoms. He asked me right away if I had been consuming any sugars. And unfortunately I had. It is so important to be on a very strict sugar-free diet to eliminate bugs.

I consider *Two Feathers Healing Formula* to be one of the most potent medicines available to humankind. And I am stating that from my own experience. *Two Feather's Healing Formula* kills parasites, fungi, breaks down tumors and possesses other benefits. And it should go without saying... you absolutely MUST have a very clean, organic, vegan and sugar-free diet and lead a healthy lifestyle; otherwise no medicines will help you. There is no magic pill, my friends! YOU, not the medicine, have to take responsibility for your health. Remember, your body is able to heal itself if given the proper stimulus and favorable environment. This environment is your diet and lifestyle.

Do I recommend *Two Feathers Healing Formula?* Yes

I do. It will help to reduce loads of parasites, viruses, and other invaders in your body, which will accelerate healing.

Two Feathers Healing Formula is very potent and if you have a sensitive stomach or if you are overly acidic, you will feel burning sensations in your stomach. You need to have Aloe juice handy. As soon as you feel burning sensations, take a spoon full of Aloe juice and the burning will subside right away.

Acupuncture plus Apitherapy

While experimenting with Dr. Cowden's protocol, Dr. Zhang's protocol and all sorts of possible supplements, I was still searching for more treatments to assist my body in healing. By doing some research I discovered a treatment called *apitherapy*. Apitherapy, or "bee therapy" (from the Latin *apis* which means bee) is the medicinal use of products made by honeybees. Products of the honeybee include bee venom, honey, pollen, royal jelly, propolis, and beeswax. Some of the conditions treated (not in any special order) are: multiple sclerosis, arthritis, wounds, pain, gout, shingles, burns, tendonitis, and infections.

The ancient Greek "Father of Medicine", Hippocrates, was among the first to recognize bee venom's healing properties. Therapies utilizing these natural properties were used throughout the ancient world's prominent civilizations such as Egypt, Greece, and China. Early human paintings made by hunter-gatherers enshrine the medicinal properties of the honeybee and all it produces, suggesting that humans have used these products since the dawn of medicine. While natural remedies may have fallen out of favor, renewed scientific exploration reinforces our old intuitions regarding the potency of the bees' natural creations. Honeybee products are often recommended to keep immune systems healthy, reduce in-flammation, and promote healthy circulation.

By mixing honeybee products with essential oils, Api-therapists have rediscovered ways to use the whole hive to create medicine. Therapies include using venom (com-monly employed in "bee sting therapy") in combination with other products, such as honey and honeycomb. These products and essential oils are combined in differ-ent ways to treat many contemporary ailments.

I located a healer on Long Island that practiced Orien-tal Medicine, Homeopathy and Apitherapy. At the time, she was all booked up so I had to wait at least two months to see her. Her name was Frederique. She was a super friendly French lady. Her house was where she practiced and it had a special healing ambience.

She took the time to ask me what felt like a zillion questions. If you are familiar with Homeopathy, you probably know that the practitioner asks tons of ques-tions about you and your habits. Some of the questions sound very weird like, *"Are you afraid of thunderstorms?"* Or *"What is the weirdest thing you like to do when you are by yourself?"* That way, the homeopath understands you better and he or she is able to design a special formula that is unique to you.

Next, I was given some homeopathic pellets before I lay down for my acupuncture treatment. Suddenly I be-came really emotional and cried the whole time I was there. I was feeling so hopeless and scared again. She ac-tually asked me if I had any emotional trauma in my life during the intake. My answer, of course was, *"Yes, my biggest trauma is Lyme disease."*

I had a back and a front treatment and when the time was up, she came back to the room with a box. The box was the size of the packaging of an iPhone box. She asked me, *"Are you ready?"* She shook the box vigorously to make the "girls" angry. When I heard the angry bees' buzz, I realized that there was no way I would undergo that kind of torture. One of the bees managed to escape and it was flying all over the room making me terrified. If it was only going to be a one-time experience—yes. However, one requires at least 10 treatments to notice the difference. I have decided to skip the bees for good.

Dr. Whitmont,
Homeopathy

66The human body has been designed to resist an infinite number of changes and attacks brought about by its environment. The secret of good health lies in successful adjustment to changing stresses on the body. 99

Harry J. Johnson

After giving up on experimenting with the "girls" (bee sting therapy), I had decided to find a classical homeopath specializing in Lyme. Luckily I found Dr. Whitmont.

Dr. Whitmont is a second-generation homeopath and practicing physician in New York. He explores the complex topic of treating Lyme disease with homeopathy. Dr. Whitmont's experience as both an alternative-minded homeopath as well as a conventionally trained M.D. gives him a unique perspective not often found in the medical community.

Dr. Whitmont's treatment approach to Lyme disease involves obtaining very detailed information about his patient, e.g., a patient's constitution, physical, emotional and mental state and accompanying symptoms. This approach is totally aligned with my values and understanding of holistic treatment. I was glad to take an approach that was tailored to my unique condition and my symptoms. Homeopathy does not offer one standard protocol for treating Lyme; therapy is based upon the individual patient. Homeopathy is about augmenting the immune system to help it deal with the body's overreaction to external irritants. The other goal of homeopathic treatment, beyond immediate recovery, is helping patients to achieve a healthier state of being so that they are less likely to become ill after potential re-exposure to Lyme disease in the future.

"In many cases, Borrelia acts as an opportunistic infection, and causes symptoms only because a person's health and immunity was already inadequate due to a myriad of other causes. In such cases, simply treating the infection and eradicating it with antibiotics does nothing to prevent recurrence or relapse in the future. The antibiotics do nothing to improve health; they only deal with a crisis. A carefully selected homeopathic medicine can not only help to eradicate the infection, but can also strengthen the immune system so that a serious relapse of symptoms becomes less likely in the future.

One of the most common causes of immune deficiency is the prior use of antibiotics. Frequent antibiotic use has been associated with many health complications, including immune dysfunction, treatment-resistant infections, symptom suppression and even cancer. Even the short-term use of antibiotics weakens the immune reaction, which, paradoxically, makes one more susceptible to Borrelia and/or other Lyme-related infections." Dr. Whitmont

I was very impressed with the results I was getting with the homeopathic treatments that were carefully prescribed by Dr. Whitmont. Many of my symptoms subsided or totally disappeared for good.

Derealization

During my worst flare-ups one of the scariest symptoms was what is known as "derealization" (and often depersonalization). It is very hard to explain what I was experiencing inside of me. I felt like I was watching the whole world around me like a movie, and I was outside. It was an "out of body" experience. I had this horrible feeling inside of me that I had never experienced before in my life. Something was really off with the biochemistry in my brain and I literally felt like my soul was leaving me. Those moments were the most difficult ones. I had multiple urges to end it all for good. The only reason I did not take my life at those moments was because of my parents. They anchored me to stay in this world. And my threshold for physical and emotional pain is extremely high. But during those moments the biochemistry in my brain would switch to something abnormal; a something that I had no control over.

My best description of it is like being out of your own body watching what is going on around you. When I got it, it would be followed by high anxiety. It is a scary and strange feeling. I had feelings of being detached from others. I also had a lot of numbness. Sometimes there was a feeling of floating; like I was off balance or not grounded.

I was feeling disconnected from the world and having a sensation of unreality. The sensation could be described as if the world has become nothing more than a projection of a film. This sensation was really distressing and was making me believe that some permanent damage had been done to my brain to cause these sensations.

Usually I would develop a panic attack during those episodes and terrible unexplained anxiety. I would crawl in my bed for a couple of days until it went away. I remember my sister called me one of those days and I started crying. She asked me what was wrong and I told her I was not feeling well. Then she would say, *"So why are you crying? Just take an aspirin."* You see, people do not understand and never will unless they experience it for themselves just what it feels like to have a chronic manmade illness.

The best thing I could do was to keep reminding myself that it was the disease that was making me feel that way — it was not me. And that it would pass. There would come a day when I would feel totally calm, totally clear and totally whole.

Autohemotherapy

‚‚Healing is a matter of time, but it is sometimes also a matter of opportunity. ‚‚

Hippocrates

After having my worst derealization moments I became so eager to try more radical treatments. I had been sick for over a year and after I would see even slight improvements I would relapse again. I then decided to try autohemotherapy.

Autohemotherapy aims to give the body a new chance at fighting off illness by removing and reintroducing the patient's blood. A minimal amount of blood is drawn from the arm then injected back in through muscle tissue. This blood is said to re-stimulate the immune response, because reintroducing the blood (including substances related to the patient's illness) forces the immune system to "see" the existing pathogens in the patient's blood. Some practitioners add natural substances that they believe will help the patient recover within the blood before reinjection. Autohemotherapy can treat allergies, chronic immune deficiency, inflammation-related illnesses, diabetes, gout, and diseases of the liver, just to name a few.

Sure enough, this treatment is popular in Europe, South America, and Canada, but it is not FDA approved in the US. Therefore, I could not really find a doctor in San Diego to perform autohemotherapy on me. Luckily my roommate at that time was a Physician Assistant graduate. When I first told her about my idea she was like, *"No way!"* But then I convinced her to practice auto-hemotherapy on me. I carefully learned instructions from a legitimate source and ordered syringes online.

Our kitchen became our surgery room. Trust me; au-tohemotherapy is a pretty bloody procedure. Every time she was drawing my blood, I was about to pass out. It did not hurt that much, but the whole process of seeing a full syringe of my own blood being injected back into my body was making me sick. I have done this process a few times and after my roommate moved out I was not able to find anyone else to practice that therapy on me. People would literally run away when I explained to them what I wanted them to do. Nurses, PAs, and even doctors do not learn that in medical school, as well as many other powerful treatments. Of course they would be skeptical to do autohemotherapy on anyone, I would imagine.

Advanced Cell Training

&&*You are your own judge. The verdict is
up to you.***&&**

Astrid Alauda

I was so eager to get better that I did not know what treatment to start next. I was really scared to spend a lot of money and time on another treatment only to relapse soon after.

One day I was cleaning my apartment and found a sealed envelope older than a year-old. It said: *"Advanced Cell Training, Your body can heal itself."* I thought it was just another scam and remembered ordering that information when I first became sick, but I had never opened the package. This time I decided to try it out. I called them and asked if I could sign up... and it was meant to be! I was told that "Lyme" class was going to start in five minutes — and if I missed the first class I would have to wait another month or more for the next class! Initially they hesitated to put me in a class without having registered first, but then they let me in.

"If you have Lyme, it is not because your immune system is weak or shut down. You have Lyme because your immune system is performing poorly and in most cases ACT can help that.

Our Lyme clientele have found that their Lyme symptoms have been dramatically reduced through the Advanced Cell Training (ACT) process." Gary Blier, ACT Founder.

At the heart of the ACT program is the belief that the body can heal itself – if it performs properly. Proper bodily performance at the cellular level is a requisite for health. Improper performance is the reason for most symptoms and correcting the body's behavioral errors through a training process, is the objective for those enrolled in ACT classes.

Bodily misbehaviors as a cause of illness are most easily understood by food allergies. Good foods, such as peanuts, only "cause" symptoms when the body over reacts and "attacks" the food rather than reacting properly and absorbing it. The digestive system is certainly able to absorb food, but the appropriate response depends on the overall health of the body.

The human immune system, when it responds properly, is able to kill pathogens responsible for not only Lyme disease, but also AIDS. *Time Magazine* reported that clinicians and researchers are, *"...zeroing in on the men's individual immune responses...."* as the primary reason why some HIV carriers don't get sick. If the responses of the human body can be positively influenced, then good food and microorganisms don't have to cause symptoms. Dis-ease can be averted. What methods does ACT employ to influence the body's behavior?

ACT uses intent and prayer plus the senses – sight, sound, touch, and focus through meditation – to reach the functional intelligence of the body. Words (called codes) that are read by the client might be germane to the pathogens at play, i.e., Borrelia strain 1 – 800, Bartonella strain 1 – 900, Mycoplasma strain 1 – 70. These are pathogens discovered by science, which may be in a Lyme victim's body.

Then the client may be asked to look at a picture of the creatures, while pressing a sore inflamed spot on a muscle or joint tissue where the pathogen are likely attacking. Music is played to assist in extended focus or meditation is performed in the hopes that the body will "recognize the errors" and therefore correct them. Gary Blier, founder of the ACT process, instituted prayer after realizing a number of double blind studies indicated the results surpassed medical placebo. Mr. Blier believes that since there is no harm in any of the processes used; why not do everything possible to try to influence the body's behaviors?

Gary Blier states that ACT is a, *"behavioral modification program for the autonomic systems of the body responsible for maintaining health and well-being."* The whole healing process with ACT was very interesting. First off, you create a chart of your top 10 worst symptoms, and every single week you rate them from 0 to 10; 0 = no symptom, 10 = worst. Sure enough, I started noticing differences in all my symptoms — they decreased. And I know it was not a placebo effect because we had over 40 people in my class, and 90% of them reported improvements at every single class! I had no idea how this process worked but all I knew was that it was working for me! Again, I was not cured overnight, but I was improving. And I highly recommend rating your symptoms weekly or even daily. When you are sick for an extended period of time, like months or even years, you slowly lose hope and think that nothing is helping you. But when you rate your symptoms, even if you are still sick, your symptoms might be at a "six" and just four months earlier they were at a "10!" Big difference!

I am the kind of person who needs to know all the answers and figure out how stuff works. You guessed it — I packed my suitcase and flew to Boston in December

2010. Oh my! After living in sunny San Diego's steady climate of 75-80 degrees, Boston weather was cruel. It was not just cold, it was snowing heavily. Don't get me wrong, I love snow but not when I did not have winter clothes and when I needed to drive a rental car in the middle of nowhere (ACT office is in Greenwich, RI. Don't forget, I am a New Yorker, so Greenwich did look like 'the middle of nowhere' to me).

By the way, Gary is booked for private consultations six months in advance. It did NOT stop me! I called the office from Boston and told them, *"I am in Boston and I am coming tomorrow to see Gary."* The office staff squeezed me in between classes.

I sat in on a 'live' class this time and after it was done I had a private session with Gary. He is a very interesting and unusual man. (What ordinary man could come up with such an amazing technique to train your immune system?!)

I had been with ACT for nine months and I was about 85% recovered. (Again, I have to note though that there is no magic and overnight cure! I was eating a very clean vegan diet. I was also exercising, practicing hot yoga, going to the sauna, and doing all kinds of spiritual work.)

In the summer of June 2011, I flew to Boston again to see Gary for another private session — because "good enough" is NOT good enough for me!

The moral of this story is... YOU have to make things happen! Yes, I was still sick and nervous about going to the East coast from the West coast, without even a scheduled appointment. But I did not let doubt stop me. I packed and took off. My health is my #1 priority. No excuses! No procrastination!

What are you waiting for? If not now, then when? And if not you, then who? I really encourage you, my friends, to take FULL RESPONSIBILITY for your health and step up! I know that you are probably low on finances, you have no energy, you are in pain, and you are unable to think straight because of constant brain fog. I've been there, I know it's hard! But you are stronger than you think! Stop feeling pity for yourself and start taking actions! Maybe this step will change your life!

I kind of already know there are many "nay sayers" when it comes to ACT. I get it, I was just like you. I wanted a "proven" method. Apparently, there are many "proven" and "approved" methods. One of my favorite sayings is, *"FDA approved – side effects guaranteed!"* Just for you skeptics — here is the ACT chart of my symptoms. As you can see, my symptoms were decreasing significantly each week!

Week	1	2	3	4	5	6	7	8	9	10	11	12
Brain Fog	10	7	2	3	1	3	1	0	1	1	1	1
Fatigue	10	7	2	3	2	5	3	0	2	2	1	3
Facial Twitch	9	6	3	4	3	5	2	2	2	2	2	2
Headache	7	3	0	2	3	2	0	1	0	2	1	3
Heartache	3	2	0	0	0	0	0	0	0	4	0	1
Muscle ache	3	1	1	4	2	2	2	1	1	2	1	2
Numbness	5	0	0	3	1	2	2	0	2	1	2	3
Depression	6	2	1	2	1	2	1	0	0	1	1	4
Skin Rash	0	5	5	0	0	0	0	0	1	0	0	0
Sound Sensitivity	3	3	3	3	3	4	2	1	2	1	1	1
Joint Pain	6	0	0	0	0	0	0	0	0	0	0	1
Panic attack	9	0	0	0	0	0	0	0	0	0	0	0
Ear ache	1	2	1	0	1	1	0	0	0	0	1	0

My Experience with a Rife Machine

66Conventional medicine is a collection of unproven prescriptions the results which, taken collectively are more fatal than useful to mankind. 99

Napoleon Bonaparte

A few months later after I started Advanced Cell Training classes, I had decided to get a Rife machine. Even though I saw improvements with my symptoms with ACT, I wanted to treat my symptoms even more aggressively, so I chose to invest in Rife. Actually I really wanted to buy my own Ondamed machine, but since it costs $25, 000, I was not able to afford one. I started researching all kinds of Rife models, types, and frequencies. I went to different forums to read reviews of different models and makes. While researching Rife equipment I came across the work of Dr. Sutherland.

His "Frequency Foundation" exposes patients to ultra-low frequency bands online, so that they can be treated anywhere in the world. Dr. Sutherland lectures in many cities in the EU and the US, so the mobility of treatments is a relief for patients. The technology employed by the "Frequency Foundation" resembles technology used to communicate with submarines through the earth and was originally developed by the Department of Defense. This history suggests that the online treatments are just as effective as in-person ones. The broadcasts can be extremely useful for patients.

So I contacted Dr. Sutherland and sent him my pictures immediately. He started running frequencies for me remotely. I was working with him for about two months, but I still had my symptoms. Dr. Sutherland was a little surprised that my case was so stubborn. So he continued working with me without even charging me anymore. A few weeks later I decided to purchase my own device; F165 and SC-1(the transmitter that allows you to send frequencies remotely).

I am very confident that Rife machines are extremely powerful in killing pathogens.

Dr. Royal Rife discovered he could use specific electro-magnetic frequencies to kill a bacteria or viruses without causing damage to the surrounding tissue. The Rife machines utilize the Law of Resonance and produce possible health benefits for varied diseases, both chronic and infectious. Though the first Rife machines were used on diseases such as tuberculosis, arthritis, and ulcers, it's more commonly known for its use on cancer, described by authors such as Barry Lynes in the book, *The Cancer Cure that Worked!*

The particular frequencies that Rife machines use cause bacteria and viruses to break apart. Abnormal electrical patterns may be responsible for illness, and Rife machines can set right many electrical imbalances while strengthening the immune system. Some people believe that Rife machines encourage the regeneration of cells, and cause tumors and cancers to "overheat and die."

Rife machines are not FDA approved. The FDA won't approve this technology for one main reason… **profits**. It cuts too much into their business. This technology kills pathogens and solves the problem. The FDA just wants to treat, not solve.

Even though I am pretty good with technology, I had a hard time operating the device and running those frequencies. I used my Rife machine for about two months and then I gave it away. At the same time, I was listening to my ACT classes, taking immune supporting herbs, and applying all the lifestyle changes I will describe in the second part of this book. So I felt like I was doing enough and my intuition pretty much "told me" that I did not really need Rife to recover.

I do not consider myself a good candidate to make any additional positive or negative claims about Rife machines; I simply did not have enough exposure to the frequencies. If you do decide to go ahead and get a Rife machine, I would definitely recommend F165 and SC-1 since it remotely sends out frequencies to you 24/7.

MMS – Miracle Mineral Solution

66*To array a man's will against his sickness is the supreme art of medicine.* 99

Henry Ward Beecher

About every six weeks I would go through very bad flare ups even when I was already getting better. One time, my flare up got so bad that I started panicking again. I was experiencing random pains, heartache, palpitations, headaches, extreme brain fog, fatigue, anxiety and derealization. I remember a friend of mine called me and said that she had something for me that I *must* try. I drove by and picked up MMS from her. I had known about MMS for a long time but I was a bit skeptical of taking it because it contains chemicals.

The MMS product and protocol was developed by Jim Humble, a gold miner and metallurgist, on an expedition into the jungles of Central America, looking for gold. It was a response to a need to help two members of his expedition who came down with malaria. They were more than two days away, through heavy jungle, from reaching the next mine. After many years of experience, Humble always carried a liquid concoction with him on these types of expeditions. This mixture, which was often referred to as "stabilized oxygen," is really sodium chlorite (NaClO2). The purpose of this solution is to make local water potable. Facing the possibility of a quick loss of life, he gave it to the stricken men. To everyone's amazement, they were both well within a few hours. That sure seemed like a miracle (as well as a huge relief), but Humble wanted to better understand what had just happened.

He ultimately discovered that chlorine dioxide, not oxygen, caused his expedition's miraculous recovery. After further investigation, he decided to use a higher concentration of social chlorite in his formula to increase the overall amount of chlorine dioxide. Use of this formula has helped thousands of people suffering from malaria, hepatitis, cancer, and AIDS to rid themselves of these diseases altogether.

After doing some research online for MMS, I had decided to give it a try. I was following the instructions and increasing the dosage every day. It did not make me sick or nauseated. The odor was pretty strong but manageable. I was taking MMS regularly for about three weeks without any side effects or noticeable results. However after three weeks, MMS gave me an upset stomach and I was not able to tolerate it anymore. I think MMS reduced significant amounts of bacteria and parasite loads for me, which was good.

"Gu Syndrome" - Demons of the Body & Mind

66He who has health, has hope; and he who has hope, has everything. 99

Arabian Proverb

Soon after I had stopped experimenting with MMS, I received an e-mail from a dear friend of mine:

"Hi Katrina,

Something wonderful happened! I was at a lecture by Heiner Fruehauf about Gu syndrome at PCOM last night. It is clear that he has the cure for Lyme! I need to talk to you about this since it's too long to elaborate on email.

Lai San."

Can you imagine my excitement after receiving this e-mail?! I began to carefully read all I could about "Gu syndrome" and was very impressed with how Dr. Fruehauf explains it and his approach to treat it.

Dr. Fruehauf's formulas reflect a unique approach to

the difficult and recalcitrant problem of chronic inflammatory disease. It is based on the Qing dynasty remedy Jiajian Su He Tang (Perilla and Mint Decoction Modified), and represents a time-honored solution for the important clinical phenomenon of "Brain Gu Syndrome" (literally means Demons of the Body & Mind): treatment resistant diseases caused by viral and spirochetal infections of the nervous system (such as chronic herpes, Lyme disease, babesiosis, bartonellosis, ehrlichiosis, and rickettsia). This formula aims to not only counteract pathogens, but also to treat terrain issues associated with various deficiencies in the patient's qi, yin, and blood.

If you look at the "Indications", you can see all the Lyme symptoms:

- Chronic debilitating joint and muscle pain (cyclical); permanent state of exhaustion

- Chronic flu-like symptoms; chronic headaches (cyclical), brain fog

- Restlessness, anxiety, insomnia; sensation of "possession" ("I want my life back")

- Grimy and stubborn tongue coating; weak (yet occasionally aggravated or tight) pulse

You cannot buy this formula without an herbalist prescription. Since I was an Oriental medicine student, I was able to "prescribe" it to myself. I was using this formula for a few months with much success. Consult your acupuncturist or an herbalist to see if this formula for "Gu syndrome" might be right for you.

You can learn more about Dr. Fruehauf's formulas at: http://www.classicalpearls.org/

Chemtrails: What in the world are they spraying?

After my recovery I would still get some Lyme-like symptoms such as brain fog and fatigue. I was not sure if I still had Lyme or if I had neurotoxins in my blood that were making me tired.

Sometimes the brain fog got really bad; I would forget to do something important, or I would lose my keys, or leave my wallet somewhere. Once I was driving in downtown LA on an early Sunday morning. The roads were empty, but it was heavily raining and foggy. The visibility was horrible and my brain fog did not help. All I remember is that I turned my head and saw a car, only a few feet away and driving at full speed, coming in my direction. I tried to escape and a second later I felt a crash of another car into mine. My car was spinning 360 degrees and ended up about 150 feet away. I was in total shock. I had no idea what had just happened, and I was behaving weird... the first thing I did was to start collecting almonds that had spread out all over my car due to the impact. Only after this did I get out of my car and realize I was in a car accident. Thank God I was not injured; I probably had Angels watching over me, because my car was a mess and it had to be in a body shop for repair for almost two months.

Luckily I had met a girl that told me about Dr. Donald Monus. Dr. Monus is a biochemical inventor and disease researcher with over 25 years of experience in all forms of disease and natural cures. His work has been referenced in medical journals and has earned him a place in the international publication of, *Who's Who in America.*

Dr. Monus is one of the best scientists who diagnoses by live blood analysis. Unlike many naturopaths that use live blood analysis for analyzing the pH level of the blood, Dr. Monus is able to recognize parasites, viruses, bacteria, mycoplasma, fungi, and other foreign invaders in one's blood. I highly recommend his book, *What's Killing You and What To Do About It!*

Dr. Monus is located in Largo, Florida. As you've already learned about me, the distance of thousands of miles did not stop me from seeing him. I flew to Florida just to meet Dr. Monus and discover what was making me sick.

First Dr. Monus checked my blood pressure. However not as a conventional doctor on one side, he checked my blood pressure several times on my both arms and explained that my heart was weak. He could tell this because of the significant difference in the readings. Then he poked my finger and said, *"In about five minutes you will know exactly what's making you sick."* To say I was very anxious is an understatement.

Dr. Monus looked into his super powerful dark field microscope and said, *"A-ha."* He showed me my blood on his computer screen and explained what he saw. He confirmed that I did not have Lyme; however, I had "aluminum chemtrail crystals" in my blood that contains all kinds of viruses, parasites, and mycoplasma.

For those of you who do not know, over the past decade and more, long white trails emanating from jet planes have been seen lingering in the skies all over the planet, often expanding and merging to form vast swathes of artificial cloud cover.

These trails are clearly not water vapor contrails, which evaporate after several minutes. They remain overhead for long extended periods of time, often culminating in strange grid like formations.

Chemtrails are loaded with heavy metal toxins that have been measured in the water and air at several different locations. And now these toxins are showing up at high levels in blood samples from regular folks who have been ill while living in "chemtrailed" areas.

Aluminum, barium, and strontium are found with high levels in all those samples. They are invisible yet are found in water and air samples at ground levels; this means they are infesting plant life and water supplies while we breathe them into our lungs. Breathing in toxins bypasses a considerable amount of our immune systems.

An Arizona resident recently collected certified medical blood test documents from seriously ill Arizonians and sent them to various State and Federal elected officials demanding an investigation. The blood sample documents showed extremely high amounts of either barium or aluminum or both. None of those people worked or had worked with hazardous materials. Some were retired.

Observe the difference between contrails and chemtrails with open eyes and an open mind. Research the internet and observe satellite photos of crisscrossing trails. Read about the established flight logs and established commercial aircraft routes that differ from those chemtrail patterns. Use the internet for more information. Watch the documentary titled, *What in the World are They Spraying?*

Taking care of yourself and your family is the first priority. You should increase heavy metal detox protocols and consume more foods that protect you from heavy metals.

"GeoEngineers Propose Atmospheric GeoEngineering to Control Climate by Spraying 10 – 20 Million Tons of Aluminum Particles Per Year into the Stratosphere. – February 20, 2010

Aluminum, Barium, Manganese, Thorium, Nickel and many other TOXIC HEAVY METALS at levels 100's of times over the Maximum Limit for human exposure. Copies of Lab Results showing data for 2008 & 2009 are available at Arizona SkyWatch."

Do you have flu-like symptoms, malaise, respiratory problems, or immune problems? Have these appeared in the past few years . . . seemingly out of nowhere?

If so, you may be a victim of chemtrails. Chemtrails spraying is going on around the world around the clock.

Many people have developed strange symptoms and chronic health problems following the spraying as the various constituents of the Chemtrails have fallen to earth.

These constituents have been particularly identified as barium and mycoplasmas. Whether the mycoplasmas are part of the original spraying or become attached to the particulate matter of the Chemtrails is unknown.

Did You Know?

Washington reporter Mike Blair wrote that what has been dubbed, *"chemtrails is actually anti-bacteriological warfare chemicals being tested by the federal government."*

It has been reported that this program gained its legality from US Code Title 50, Section 1520, which gives the Secretary of Defense authority to order testing *"involving the use of a chemical agent or biological agent on a civilian population"* for research purposes.

Chemtrails are clearly seen.

In the bill Chemtrails are listed as an, *"exotic weapons system."*

Are your health problems caused by germ warfare or government experiments?

Samples from these Chemtrails were analyzed by a facility in Victoria, British Columbia, which is licensed by the U. S. Environmental Protection Agency (EPA) and found to contain in addition to JP-8 jet fuel (possibly the carrier medium which contains the additive ethylene dibromide, banned as a pesticide due to causing severe respiratory reactions even at low levels) numerous pathogens, and disease causing agents.

I encourage you to go to www.curezone.com and search "Chemtrail disease". The information will blow your mind!

Brain Fog and How to Deal with It

Just as many of you with neurological Lyme, one of the worst symptoms of mine was brain fog (always accompanied by fatigue). As I mentioned earlier, I would forget my own phone number and I would not be able to complete simple tasks. Again, during one of the worst episodes of brain fog I was involved in a major car accident. Brain fog is caused by a load of neurotoxins that Lyme produces as well as by other factors.

Causes of Brain Fog range from garden variety to medically obscure, including: Adrenal fatigues syndrome, insomnia, Chronic Fatigue Syndrome, nutritional deficiency, Candidiasis, Fibromyalgia and MS, chronic viral infections (such as Lyme disease), parasitic organisms, heavy metal toxicity, circulatory problems, uncontrolled blood sugar, overuse of artificial sweeteners and MSG, allergies and food intolerance, leaky gut, side effects of medicine, constipation, menopause, and even sick building syndrome. Each of these causes involves the diversion of bodily resources from the goal of maintaining wellness to dealing with an internal emergency. In the case of the nutrition-related disorders, your energy is going to supplement what you should be getting, while in the case of allergies and chronic viral infections your resources are tied up in chronic inner battles.

There are a number of methods that can be used to help relieve brain fog. Brain fog is a term to describe impaired or slowed thought, and is a common symptom experienced by individuals with adrenal fatigue. There are many brain fog relief remedies to help improve energy levels, mental clarity and brain function.

By making sure to keep yourself properly nourished, you can limit the effects of brain fog on your body. Eat plenty of green leafy vegetables, wholegrain foods, and foods that contain Omega-3 fatty acids. Eating well (and taking supplements) makes sure that you have the nutrients and minerals you need to keep your energy up, so that you divert fewer resources to basic functioning and can feel more aware and alive. Natural supplements known to reduce brain fog are multivitamins and B12 supplements. Ginkgo Biloba may reduce brain fog by allowing improved circulation and oxygen to the brain. "Pinella" from Nutramix is great, and some people swear by turmeric.

Drinking lots of water with lemon also helps by flushing out toxins and further reducing the amount of energy you have to use for basic functioning.

As always, physical activity is a must. By increasing oxygen flow, boosting energy, and improving circulation, exercise is a crucial factor in keeping your brain healthy. If you begin regular physical activity, you will see improvements in your cognitive abilities and mood thanks to the additional production of serotonin and endorphins. Another benefit of exercise: you might sleep better! Sleeping well is difficult for many of us, but getting eight hours of sleep every night can reduce brain fog and increase your cognitive abilities. As you keep improving your health, you will find sleeping easier and experience less brain fog.

For me personally, the best relief from brain fog was to detox physically by sweating. No matter how tired and foggy I felt, I would go for a run and I always felt better even for a bit. The best brain fog elevation treatment for me was hyperthermia, i.e. sauna or even better – hot yoga. (I do not recommend a steam room just because municipal water is chlorinated and while in a steam room you will inhale too much toxic chlorine). As soon as I started sweating, loads of toxins left my body through sweat and I felt better immediately. Also, taking activated charcoal, coffee enemas, and drinking plenty of water with lemon worked for me.

REAL CASES:

I am having the worst brain fog. I feel like a cotton ball has replaced my brain. Today is soooo much worse. I can't remember what I'm saying when I'm half way through saying it!! I have had to stop and have the kids remind me what we are even talking about... I can't follow a conversation or attempt to hold one. My head feels pressurized and I feel shaky. I literally feel like I'm lost. Everything feels so strange. I don't know what I'm doing....

ॐ ॐ

I really really struggled in college. I was used to putting in a certain amount of effort and achieving good results. When Lyme hit me in college, I couldn't grasp ANYTHING at all. It took 10 times the amount of time to memorize something simple... then I would forget so quickly.

ॐ ॐ

My experience with brain fog is, forgetting things even after looking at a list seconds before. Head feels heavy, confu-

sion, can't multi-task for nothing, feelings of not being in my own body, like I am watching what's going on from behind myself. Can't recall certain words or phrases.

My brain fog was disorientation, forgetfulness and I always wanted to tell people, 'I don't feel like I am here right now.'

For me, the best way I can describe it, is it feels like there is a fog or mist around every thought, memory, or any piece of information I am trying to retrieve in my head. If I sit there long enough trying to remember something, I can retrieve the information I'm thinking about, but sometimes I can't and just go blank or give up trying.

Also my short term memory is pretty bad. I can read a paragraph of information and literally 5 seconds later I remember 0% of it.

I am now a firm believer in the benefits of Apple Cider Vinegar. For the past 6 months I have been suffering from extreme fatigue, and do not know why. I've been to too many doctors and not one can tell me why. I started taking ACV on a regular basis (3T per day) for the past 2 week. I can't even explain how much better I feel...it has given me my life back after 6 months of suffering. I still do not know what exactly is causing the fatigue, but I no longer have it! I would recommend this to everyone! I feel great, no more brain fog, fatigue, sore throat and my headaches are GONE. I finally feel normal again!

07/28/2007: Ted from Bangkok, Thailand: "Remedies for brain fog is a long one, but to keep it really short, alkalizing is

the basic as alkalization dilates the capillaries, which includes the brain.

Certain infections, yeast, candida can initiate a brain fog too, as much as mycoplasma, mycobacterium and other microbial overload. The one interesting aspect of alkalization is these microorganisms don't survive well in alkaline and high oxygen environments.

There are certain other supplements that have high antifungals (which causes brain fogs), and heavy metal accumulation can also lead to brain fog (when you take antibiotics, heavy metal accumulates), and even in the event of vaccination (mycoplasma they are living, exist causing brain fog, but also the mercury and the aluminum they added). Therefore, molybdenum and boron (from borax) have antifungal properties too. Molybdenum is a well know antioxidant, at least for me, which exists in superoxide dismutase along with copper and zinc also."

If you haven't yet seen this article on Earth Clinic (www. earthclinic.com), we suggest you take a moment to read Jason Uttley's brilliant article **Chronic Fluoride Poisoning. One of the more common side effects of CFP is brain fog.**

Family/ Friends Drama

> **66**To forgive is the highest, most beautiful
> form of love. In return, you will receive
> untold peace and happiness. **99**
>
> Dr. Robert Muller

"Oh, but you look good!" they say, thinking they're making you feel better. Inside, your stomach grows tight; you inwardly cringe, and fight the urge to scream. 'On No! Not this again!' you think. Welcome to the world of Invisible Chronic Illness. This is a hard world to live in, one in which you're positive no one could possibly understand how hard it is to live like this. Well, I'm writing this to tell you that someone does understand. In fact, anyone living with Lyme disease probably understands. Your body hurts, fatigue seems like such an ineffectual word for what you're feeling, you constantly struggle to find words you want to express, and yet, "You LOOK great!" (Geri Fosseen, Director, of the Iowa Lyme Disease Foundation, Melissa Kaplan's Chronic Neuroimmune Diseases Information on CFS, FM, MCS, Lyme Disease, Thyroid, and more)

The most scary and difficult part on my healing

journey was the feeling of loneliness and sadness; being abandoned by my own family members. I was praying to God every day to forgive them and to let go. I was repeating affirmations every single day that I forgave myself and I forgave them. But those were only words — empty words. Deep down in my heart I had grief that like a black massive stone was dragging me down under the water. I was brokenhearted and hopeless.

It all started when I had first become sick; when my sister and other family members abandoned me when I was asking for help. And I did not really ask for much... I asked once for someone to escort me to Montreal when my face was paralyzed and I was extremely sick, but no family member did. Remember, I was always "Miss Independent" so I've never asked for anything else after that. But I was really expecting some phone calls. I needed support like never before. I needed someone checking in on me once in a while. No one did....

Unfortunately my health was declining rapidly. About two months after I was diagnosed, I start "losing it." I was not able to take care of myself anymore; I was scared, terrified, and devastated. My last hope was for my sister and my brother-in-law to step up and help me. Actually, my last hope was my brother-in-law since my sister was questioning me as to whether I even had Lyme. This is the letter I sent to my brother-in-law.

S, I am writing to you because I am stuck with my health-issue and I don't know where to go. When I talk to T, she tells me that it's in my head and today she was even asking if I am sure I have Lyme. I was partially paralyzed, I was in the ER with crazy symptoms, I am experiencing horrible symptoms every day, I am not insane to fabricate all of this! If you doubt also, I can continue... I went to the best MD's in NYC; they all agreed I have Lyme. The biofeedback I am doing now shows Lyme and co-infections.

Even though I am not a fan of conventional meds, I was on antibiotics for 2 months! It did not help. I am taking 50 tablets of herbs every day and I don't know if they work...

Every morning I wake just to get some new symptoms. I had inflammation in my body that caused horrible muscle and joint pain, I was still dealing with that with an attitude that it's a healing crisis and it's going to get only better. I have fatigue and low energy every day, I manage to go to school, but I am not able to work anymore ...   Now I am afraid it's getting worse, because it's affecting my brain. A week ago I could not find my car and called 911, I was sure the spot where I parked it was empty; I thought the car was stolen. I found it on the next block. Yesterday I was not able to recall my own phone number (I know, T told me it happens to everyone, but it does not! I know when I am normal and when I am not) Today I was not able to study, I had brain fog all day long, and on a test in school I was not able to remember anything I studied for the past year. Lyme makes me extremely anxious and paranoid.

I am getting biofeedback treatments which I feel is helping me, but I cannot afford more than 2 a week, I am getting acupuncture, taking all possible herbs, but I don't know if I will ever get better.

I did so much research and, "as most, sufferers know, there really isn't much real science as it pertains to the treatment of Lyme disease. Many 'LLMDs' (Lyme literate medical doctors) disagree about how to treat patients, and no LLMD I have heard of has astonishing success. With Lyme disease, it's almost always hit-and-miss. Maybe 'Lyme Literate Medical Doctors' should be renamed: 'Doctors Desperately Fighting a Losing Battle.' "

So, the reason I write to you, because you are the most adequate person in a family (I can't even talk to my parents, if I *tell them I am sick, they get totally paranoid, if I tell them I am ok, they are telling me to stop treatments because people are just trying to get $$ out of me) and I can't think for myself anymore, I am slowly losing my mind.*

S, if you could think of anything that I should do please let me know. I am a total mess now.

Love you guys T+ N :-)

Katrina

And guess what? I did not hear from my brother-in-law for several days, and then he finally called and offered for me to come and stay at their house. I could hear total disbelief in his voice about my illness. That was the last time I have ever asked them for help.

Later, I had shipped them the DVD called, *Under Our Skin* in the hope that they would learn more about the disease and horror I was going through. My sister did not even watch it.

It took me a long time, close to two years to let go of my feelings towards my family. I knew that any grief or resentment in my heart would delay my healing. I was meditating and practicing forgiveness exercises by myself as well as I had a healer working on me addressing "forgiveness" issues.

Forgiving others and even forgiving ourselves is not always easy. In fact, how do you forgive someone who has hurt you? How do you forgive yourself for regrets that you have? The truth is, even when we want to engage in the process of forgiving others or ourselves in our mind, we don't always know how to let go from our heart.

I remember exactly the moment when I genuinely and

for good finally forgave my sister. I was attending Tony Robbins seminar in Fort Lauderdale, FL in June 2011. I was so occupied with the workshops we had there that I even forgot I once had Lyme. At one of the workshops we had learned about the kind of chiropractic adjustments when the practitioner is not using any pressure but only energy to adjust a patient. As an acupuncturist and health practitioner I became really interested in learning more about that technique. That evening I noticed a guy in our group that happened to be a chiropractor. I asked him if he knew about that method and if he could adjust me. He agreed and we went outside by the hotel pool. His energy was just amazing. We started talking and I do not know how and why but I told him my entire life story, crying my eyes out. When I told him about my resentment to my sister, he guided me through a healing process. I did not know it would have such a significant impact on my life. I felt like that black stone down in my heart disappeared and light and love took its place. It felt really liberating. I am so grateful for that experience! His name was David. (And if he is reading this book I want him to know that I will cherish that moment in my heart for the rest of my life!)

I would like to offer you a "forgiveness" exercise that hopefully will clear out any and all negative emotions you may have towards your friends and family.

To do this forgiveness exercise, choose a quiet, comfortable place where you will be free from distractions. Give yourself at least an hour to complete this exercise from beginning to end. You will need some paper and a pen.

Don't hold to anger, hurt, or pain. They steal your energy and keep you from love. Leo Buscaglia

1. Make a list of names.

To begin the process of forgiving others, write down the name of every person (even if they are no longer living) who has irritated or offended you in some way. If that hurt or upset is still with you, their name goes on the list.

You will be amazed at the memories that come to you. People may come to your mind that you haven't thought about in years.

Also, be sure to put your own name on the list to forgive yourself for regrets that you may have. Keep writing names until you can't think of anyone else to add.

2. Spend some time forgiving each person on your list.

Look at the first name on your list, close your eyes and then hold the image of each person in your mind and tell him or her, *"I forgive you and I release you. I hold no unforgiveness back. My forgiveness for you is total. I am free and you are free."*

Once you say the affirmation, feel the truth of these words in your body. Feel how good it feels to let go. Continue to do this with each person on your list.

3. Notice how you feel and write about your experience.

After you "speak to" the last person, pause for a moment to notice how you feel. You can write about your experience if you wish.

4. Express and feel your gratitude.

If you asked for spiritual assistance, this is a good time to give thanks for the support that you received.

To end this session of forgiving others and forgiving yourself, close your eyes and bring your awareness into your heart, allow your heart to fill with gratitude for the releasing that took place.

When I look back at those suffering years, it makes me really sad to remember that no one could relate to how hard mentally and physically it was for me to live with a chronic, "invisible" illness. It was not possible to explain to friends, they thought I was totally fabricating stuff. It was not possible to explain to family. It was not possible to explain even to doctors! And now I am trying to look at the whole situation from a different perspective. Just try to remember yourself before you got sick. Remember yourself when you were happy and healthy. If someone told you about Lyme symptoms you would probably not be able to relate to them.

I remember when I first was diagnosed; I was herxing a lot from antibiotics and was really sick overall. I was still going to school part time. (I was studying Oriental medicine) And all of my professors knew I was dealing with Lyme yet, none of them could relate. They would not let me take a quiz if I arrived to class 10 minutes late. (By their policy you cannot take a quiz if you were late) And for me it was such a challenge to just leave my bed and make it to school, because of chronic fatigue, pain, weakness and exhaustion. It was challenging to take a shower, not to mention to make it almost on time for a class. But they could not understand how sick I really was. They would treat me like Lyme was a common cold and that I was just lazy. One professor gave me a "C" just because I was not "proactive" enough in my clinic shift. And that professor was an infectious disease specialist! And for me it was such an accomplishment just to make it through my shift and serve patients without anybody guessing that I was sicker than any of my patients! Then I transferred to the San Diego campus because I was not able to handle the hectic lifestyle of living in New York City anymore. During my second semester at the San Diego school, I "failed" my clinic shift because I missed my shift without a doctor's note. I went to the clinic director, clinic manager, school director, dean, and other authorities, to explain that I was dealing with Lyme and that I missed my shift (which I made up within a few days) because I had an appointment with a healer on the East Coast. Because my healer was not an MD, he could not give me an "excuse". It took me numerous "board" meetings and letters to different school authorities to "pass" my clinic shift. So can you imagine if even doctors and healers in medical school think you are fabricating stuff, it is very hard for "normal" people to relate and understand what we are going through...?

One time I was visiting my sis in Memphis. And she got upset at me that I was sleeping till noon, and that I took off to a health food store to get my wheatgrass shot instead of spending time with the family. I wished they could understand that extreme fatigue and longer hours of sleep were not a luxury for me; I would trade anything to be healthy. And I wish I could have gone with my little niece for an ice-cream instead of driving across town looking for a juice bar and wheatgrass.

Letters from those with "Invisible" Illnesses

❝Just because you're not sick doesn't mean you're healthy. ❞

Unknown

"Dear Friends and Family,

I look normal, I am not. Don't let my outward appearance fool you; I am in pain and I am exhausted. I am not the same person I was a year ago or two years ago for that matter. I look healthy, I am not.

My condition changes from day to day, sometimes even hour to hour. Today I may be able to go to work; tomorrow I may not be able to get out of bed. This week I feel horrible. Next week I may feel good. I want to do all the things I used to; go to the mall for the day, work in my yard, visit friends and relatives, keep my house in order, but I may not be capable of it.

If I say 'not today,' or 'I can't come,' please understand and accept this for what it is, which is not an excuse. It is a reason. I don't enjoy my limitations, I hate them. I may be able to do *today what you want me to do, but I know without a doubt, that I will suffer an incredible amount of pain later; therefore I must say 'no'. Sometimes I feel overwhelmed with the things that have to be done around the house. I'm afraid to ask for help because I feel like you don't think I "really" need it; that if I would just get up and do it, things would get done. Lyme disease doesn't work that way. I am not lazy, I just hurt and am exhausted.*

I don't feel sorry for myself, why should I? Things don't always work out the way you'd like them to... this is one of those times. I can live with who I am now. I may not enjoy each day as much as I used to, but I still live for each day and embrace whatever I can get out of life. Pain is my companion, but pain is not me.

The hard part is if you cannot accept me for who I am now, I am sorry for you. I won't waste time chasing after your friendships, approval, love or understanding. To preserve myself and state-of-mind, I have to be selfish. If you cannot accept that I may not call you every day, go places with you, or visit you then do me a favor and let's part ways quietly with no ill feelings.

My life is going in a new direction and for me that might not be a bad thing. If the changes I have gone through disturb you, hold your criticism. I don't need it. I don't want it.

Life deals us all a bad hand occasionally. This is the hand I have been dealt and I intend to play it out.

It happened... I accepted it... I hope you can too."

Anonymous

⚬ ⚬

"Hi all. I'm very newly diagnosed and just started treatment. Can anyone give me tips on how to explain Lyme to my husband, friends and family members? Unless you have Lyme, I think it's very difficult to truly understand it.

For example, my husband doesn't understand why I can't go grocery shopping, do several loads of laundry and take a trip to Costco in one day. The problem may be that I push myself way too much, because I feel guilty about being sick, but then I give him the impression that I'm actually capable of doing these things. When really, I should be pacing myself and resting more.

So, does anyone have any ideas on how to convey the disabling effects of this disease to others?"

Anonymous

◡ ◡

"But You Don't LOOK Sick....

One of the hardest parts of having Lyme disease is that every single aspect of my disease is completely naked to the visible eye. It's surreal that there are no outward signs of the pain going on behind the scenes inside my body. If I don't tell someone I am sick, they have no idea. Even my closest friends have difficulty gauging how I'm feeling unless I verbalize it.

One thing that always throws me off is the comment, 'You look like you're feeling great today!' While it's a blessing that I don't usually look as badly as I feel, it's incredibly jarring that my physical appearance can be so utterly incongruent with my pain levels.

Inside my body, on any given day, I'm battling dozens of symptoms that no one can see. Yet, I'm expected to function like a "normal" person, because I still look like a normal person (No comments from my brother here!). When I first came to my Lyme doctor, I had over 60 symptoms--and not a single one visible to anyone else! With treatment, we've whittled that symptom list down to a much smaller number of symptoms, *but like I said, there are still dozens. With so much going on in my body and in my life that no one can see but me, I feel so torn--after all, it's really nobody's business but my own if I'm sick, so why the need for people to know and understand Lyme disease? Simply put, doctor after doctor discredited my Lyme disease as being all in my head because I didn't/don't 'look' sick. I don't want others going through the hell that I went through to get diagnosed, but unfortunately that's exactly what is happening all across the country. "*

∽ ∽

"10 Commandments for interacting with the chronically ill:

In the realm of chronic illness, one of our more challenging tasks can be gaining support from others. As if finding a knowledgeable and caring doctor wasn't difficult enough, finding caring and supportive friends to surround ourselves with can be even more difficult. Most people are simply not capable of understanding, unless they have the misfortune of a chronic illness of their own.

How many of us have heard something along the lines of 'But you don't LOOK sick...?' It makes one wonder how a sick person is 'supposed' to look. If one were to hobble around on crutches, would their illness suddenly become more believable? Our society understands the visible, physical manifestations of illness, such as a broken bone in a cast or hair loss from chemotherapy. What many fail to grasp is the subtle, invisible manifestations of chronic illness. Symptoms such as pain, severe fatigue, and cognitive impairments are not easily visible to the average observer, which means that sufferers of chronic illness often look 'just fine'.

Our society is all about instant results - the mindset that we can just pop a magic pill and all our troubles will go away. When sufferers of a chronic illness do not quickly 'get better', we are often treated as if it were somehow our own fault. We may even be told that we are 'hypochondriacs' or that 'it's all in our head'.

Remember when you had the flu? You were exhausted, achy all over, and could hardly get out of bed. But, fortunately, the illness passed and you were back to your old self and usual activities.

Now, imagine if you had never recovered from that flu. Every day, you wake up achingly sore and as tired as if you had not slept at all. Imagine trying to go through your usual activities while feeling this way. Not only do work, school, and regular tasks of daily living become near-impossible, but so do the smaller day-to-day things that so many take for granted, such as simply washing your hair or paying the bills.

It is stressful, it is exhausting, it is depressing... and yet the chronically-ill person continues on in the face of it all.

For those of you who may have, at some point, been the perpetrator of an otherwise well-intentioned comment, please understand that our illness is just as real as that of an amputee or other 'visible' illness. To help aid those of you who wonder how to interact with a chronically ill person, allow me to present the Ten Commandments:

1. Thou Shalt Not Imply That We Are Not Truly Ill.

You will not convince us otherwise with remarks such as, 'You LOOK good,' or 'But you don't LOOK sick.' Even if you meant them as compliments, we perceive those kinds of statements as insults because they imply that you do not believe us.

2. Thou Shalt Not Imply That The Illness Can Be Easily Fixed.

People with chronic illnesses are persistent, if nothing else. We hang on, day after day. We see countless doctors, take numerous medications, do endless research, and continue hoping that the answer is just around the next corner. So please do not insult us by delivering diagnoses, remedies, or comments such as, 'Why don't you just...' or 'Have you tried...' or 'You should....' If it truly were that simple, I assure you that we would have done it already. We are sick, not stupid.

3. Thou Shalt Not Imply That We Brought This On Ourselves.

We did not choose to become ill, just as we do not choose to stay ill. Simply having a positive attitude is not going to solve our problem. One would never imply that a quadriplegic chose such a trial for themselves, or could get better 'if they really wanted to.' Please afford chronically ill patients the same respect.

4. Thou Shalt Not Insult or Argue With Our Limitations or Behaviors.

If people with chronic illnesses push ourselves too hard, we can suffer serious consequences. Most of us have developed coping mechanisms to help us survive, and it is cruel to expect us to do more than we are able. One chronically-ill woman I know was actually told, 'I wish I could have the luxury of sleeping all day.' Believe me, we would much rather be out working, playing, spending time with loved ones, participating in normal activities.

'Sleeping all day' is not a luxury for us – it is a critical necessity, one that we must take in order to protect whatever remaining health we have. Perhaps it may help to think of it in terms of being one of the medications we need to take. If you wouldn't think of denying a diabetic their insulin, then don't think of denying the sufferer of a chronic illness their critical need, whether it is a mid-day nap, avoidance of certain foods or environmental factors, or something else.

5. Thou Shalt Not Imply That You Can Relate To What We Are Going Through.

Unless you have a chronic illness of your own, you cannot

possibly understand just how much suffering is happening. Of course you want to be compassionate and want to relate to people. But when you try to do this by telling a chronically-ill person that you are always tired too, it tends to make the person feel that you are minimizing their suffering. Try saying something more along the lines of, 'This must be so hard for you,' or 'I can't imagine what you're going through.' It really does make a difference to us.

6. Thou Shalt Be Mindful Of Other Family Members.

Chronic illness doesn't just affect the person who has it, but the whole family as well. The trauma of the illness can evoke feelings of fear, depression, anger, and helplessness in all family members. The balance of family dynamics will most likely change, especially if it is a parent who is ill. The healthy spouse may end up taking on an overwhelming amount of responsibility, and even children will likely be involved in helping care for the ailing family member. Please keep these others in your thoughts as well, and make an effort to direct some special attention to them, without any mention of illness or disability.

External support from friends, neighbors, extended family, religious institutions, and support groups may help ease some of the burden.

7. Thou Shalt Acknowledge Our Efforts and Celebrate Even Our Small Successes With Us.

For the chronically ill, any day that we can accomplish a task, no matter how small, is a 'good' day! Our lives are often measured in terms of doctor's visits and lab work, and our 'success' measured by a rise in 'Natural Killer' cell counts in our blood, or actually completing an entire load of laundry in just one day. Please do not look at us as if we are joking when we share these celebratory moments with you. Celebrate with us, be happy with us, and do not kill the moment by announcing that you just completed the Ironman Triathlon in record time.

8. Thou Shalt Offer Thy Specific Help.

There are so many ways to help -- the most difficult part is usually getting a chronically-ill person to accept that help. They do not want to feel like a 'burden'. If you offer a vague, 'Call me if I can help,' the call will probably never come. But if you are sincere, consider extending offers of specific help, such as a ride to a doctor's appointment, or picking up a few groceries or the dry cleaning. These activities can be done in a way that does not add any extra burden to your own schedule. If you have to go to the grocery store for your own family, it really isn't much extra work to grab an additional loaf of bread and jug of milk. If you have to swing by the post office, getting an extra roll of stamps or mailing an additional package isn't much extra effort for you – but it can save a chronically-ill individual a lot of time, energy, and exacerbation of symptoms.

9. Thou Shalt Remember Important Events.

I'm not just talking about birthdays and Christmas. A major doctor's appointment, lab test, or new medications are all important events to the chronically-ill person. Try to sincerely ask, 'How was your appointment? How did the lab test go? How's your new medication?' The chronically-ill person will appreciate that you remembered, and that you cared enough to ask about it.

10. Thou Shalt Get To Know The Person Behind The Illness.

The illness may be a part of us, but it's not a part of who we ARE. We want to be known as more than 'that sick person'. You may discover that we have a wickedly funny sense of humor, a creative imagination, musical talents, or any number of things that better describe who we are, and what we would rather be remembered for.

Most of all, please remember that the chronically-ill person is more than worthy of love, friendship, and support. Most chronically-ill people I know are the toughest nuts I have ever met. Indeed, I have come to believe that a chronic illness is not for wimps – rather, only the toughest of the tough can continually face the struggles of life while battling a debilitating disease. That kind of grit deserves nothing less than pure respect and admiration, even from our toughest critic -- ourselves."

And now I would like to talk directly to family members. Please try to learn as much as possible about Lyme disease, so that you know what your sick family member is going through. It is so common when family refuses to believe that there is anything wrong with the sick person. He or she just looks so normal!

Family members, please read a book called, *Cure Unknown: Inside the Lyme Epidemic* by Pamela Weintraub, watch the documentary *Under Our Skin* directed by Andy Abrahams Wilson, attend Lyme conferences, and do some research on Lyme. Please accompany your loved ones to doctor appointments – at least on occasion.

Some people do not believe in Lyme disease, or they think that we are not doing enough to get well and it's our fault. It is very hard for those who have never had an "invisible" illness to understand what we are going through. Please, open your minds! Your loved ones may look totally fine, but in reality they are totally disabled by pains, agony, neurological dysfunctions, extreme fatigue and brain fog.

The biggest death rate in Lyme disease is from suicide. Please take the time to listen to your sick family member – show them you love and care about them. Help him or her do some grocery shopping, or some small things around the house, and if you can... help financially.

Success Stories

66_We've all heard about people who've exploded beyond the limitations of their conditions to become examples of the unlimited power of the human spirit._

You and I can make our lives one of these legendary inspirations, as well, simply by having courage and the awareness that we can control whatever happens in our lives. Although we cannot always control the events in our lives, we can always control our response to them, and the actions we take as a result.

If there's anything you're not happy about--in your relationships, in your health, in your career--make a decision right now about how you're going to change it immediately. **99**

Anthony Robbins

"I compare having Lyme disease to being lost at sea. You float along on the vast ocean. Sometimes you get a glimpse of the land... on good days you even get to touch the land. Then for some mysterious reason, you float back out to sea... into nothingness. I have reached the land. Some days I still drift off shore a little, but I can now always reach down and wiggle my toes in the sand... and the sand feels good"

Cheryl

When I was at the peak of my sickness, I found some videos on *YouTube* about a girl named Heather however; they were uploaded by another Lyme survivor. I have learned a lot from Heather's videos and her website. I wanted to connect with her since she became one of my heroes.

Recently I have personally met Heather (for a raw vegan lunch in Orange County, CA). Her story sounds even more dramatic and scary than it does on paper. Heather is a real fighter! She does not take "no" for an answer, that's why she is one of the warriors! And I really encourage you to join our club!

Here is her story:

"Lyme disease is a debilitating bacteria that comes from ticks carrying the disease. It has become a growing epidemic throughout the world and is grossly under diagnosed (or in my case, misdiagnosed). Due to the inability of medical experts to accurately diagnose Lyme disease, many people suffer for years without understanding what is wrong with them.

In my case, I spent years going to psychologists and psychiatrists trying to understand the cause of my anxiety, depersonalization and derealization. After being dismissed by these doctors, I found myself flat broke huddled in a corner of my apartment trembling in fear with medical bills stacked high, creditors calling me off the hook, and insurance companies refusing to pay for the medical services I had received. As I looked at myself in the mirror, I saw I was beaten down to a tiny fraction of the person I once was. I was depleted. More so, I felt dead physically, mentally, emotionally and spiritually. I had been a high functioning attorney, and now my cognitive skills were so damaged that I couldn't add and subtract numbers anymore or even read! How was I going to pay back the loans?

Abandoned by doctors after following a 30-day protocol of antibiotics, coined incurable by psychiatrists lacking knowledge of Lyme disease as the 'great imitator' of anxiety and depersonalization, unable to find a good doctor as there are very few practicing LLMD's (Lyme Literate Medical Doctors), and denied by insurance companies to pay for any of my treatments, I was forced to take my health into my own hands.

On July 1, 2009 I remember sitting in the doctor's office getting my antibiotics when I started telling the doctor that I was relapsing again. I sat in the doctor's office telling him about horrible brain fog, derealization, heart palpitations, hotness in the back of my neck, hot and cold sweats, tingling in my hands and feet, migraines and exhaustion. He said this was normal and then the nurses came into the room and wanted to take my blood. They were laughing and talking about what they were going to do for July 4th.

Tears literally began to swell up in me as I don't even remember the last time I went out with friends or had a life for that matter. They were also laughing at me because my veins were too small and it was too hard to inject me with a needle.

That drive home from the doctors was the worst day of my life. The words from my doctor that 'I might have this for the rest of my life' really made me want to drive my car off the road. If he knew how I felt he wouldn't want to live either. Thankfully I was able to drive that day because my family got tired of taking me to doctors and tired of me being sick.

A couple of weeks later it was my birthday. I was broke. I mean really broke but knew it would take a lot of money to get me out of this. I sat in my room alone on my birthday with no friends but me and a candle. I sat there holding the candle praying to God to give me money for treatments, hope and be there for me through all of this.

After I blew it out, I ran to my computer and bought myself my first birthday gift. An infrared sauna from Promolife. It was perfect because here I was sitting on my friends couch and it rolls up like a blanket. As I clicked the button to pay I literally had one eye open and was shaking - Okay I can do this. I'll just pay it off when I'm better. It's funny but I have been saying this with each treatment and have actually been able to pay it off 6 months later! Amazing the power of GOD!

That day I knew I had no choice but to seek help and get on the right track. I started talking to P. F. and seeing alternative healers. Going off antibiotics was scary for me. I won't lie. It wasn't an easy task but I just said, 'I'm dying anyway what difference does it make, let me try this for 6 months.'

Every day for 6 months now I have pretty much been my own doctor. I get up and have a routine. Routines are SO important with this. It was important for me to just keep going. Even though some days I had set backs, I would pray that what I was doing was right for my body.

Every day for the past 7 months I take vitamins in the morning, minerals and aloe. Then depending, I incorporate vitamin IV C drips, ozone water (sometimes I drink this with my vitamins), Biofeedback machines, Salt C protocol and many others including a parasite cleanse.

I can't believe that I am living again. I have dreamed of this for 4 years. Lyme has manifested itself in me in some pretty weird ways but I know everything happens for a reason and it's strange but I almost don't want to take back my Lyme. I'm so grateful today and hope my story will bring hope to people when life seems so hopeless. My dream ultimately is to have a rehabilitation center for people with Lyme to go to. It's been my dream to open up a Spa or Rehabilitation center, a place for Lymies to call home. It was everything I wanted when I was sick, alone and my family couldn't understand this disease at all.

I found comfort during those bad days by talking to other Lymies. I'm seriously crying writing this because it was just so bad and awful. Please remember no matter how bad it gets that there IS hope. You guys are my family, have saved me and I wouldn't be here today without the help from the Lyme community. God Bless You all!"

Heather Levine

You can read Heather's full story and treatment protocol at: http://www.ladderbridges.com/

The next story is written by a 19 year old who is my biggest hero. This girl went through the worst hell possible due to complications from Lyme disease, and she managed to remain strong and positive and be an example to others of how to be a warrior and never give up.

"I wasn't like most sixteen year olds. I had a blueprint of what my life was to be like in the future. I had goals that I wanted to fulfill and I knew exactly what type of woman that I wanted to grow up to be: the beauty and the brains. I wanted to go to college. I wanted to be a nurse more than anything; I wanted to be the superwoman that made sick people healthy again and who could save lives' it was my absolute passion to help people. With hard work, I wanted to buy myself a nice house. Then when the time was right, fall in love, become a wife and mother, and live happily ever after. If I worked hard enough and fought hard enough for it, I could make it all happen, but I never would have guessed that I would have to fight for my life.

I always noticed weird things happening to my body growing up. As early as ten years old, I would yawn a lot because I felt like I wasn't getting enough air. At eleven years old, I was getting dizzy spells and was being checked for brain tumors. I would always get sick with 'viruses' that would last for weeks and the same exact virus would return a month or two later. At fifteen, I noticed that I was super fatigued, even with astronomical amounts of sleep. My body craved sleep. Walking up a flight of stairs started making me dizzy and out of breath almost to the point of passing out. Schoolwork became difficult, because I could not remember what the material was. It wasn't that I was lazy or not paying attention it was to the point where I didn't know where I was going or why I was where I was at the moment. I was scared, but at the same time I didn't think anything was seriously wrong.

In the summer about a month after my sweet sixteen, I woke up in the middle of the night with a pounding headache. I actually felt my brain pulsating; it was so agonizing that I began to scream in pain. My neck was so stiff that I could not move it and my spine felt like it was on fire. My heart was skipping and fluttering. There was pain in my joints and bones' it felt like I was being stabbed all over my body with an ice pick. A trip to the emergency room was in order that night and I was scared to death.

Yet, nothing was wrong. To my dismay, I was just dehydrated, but the pain remained. I was confused as to why I was in crippling pain. I would lie in bed at night and would lie completely still. I would barely make an effort to breathe, because it hurt. 'Am I dying?' This was the only question that would race through my mind. I was old enough to understand what was happening, yet I wasn't old enough to understand why it was happening to me. There were countless nights where I would lay completely awake and feel, but pray to God that I didn't have to feel it anymore.

A week later, my walking became extremely disoriented. My knees buckled and my upper body swayed as I would carefully put one foot in front of the other. I couldn't make a connection to my legs, which felt like they had cinderblocks attached to them. The pain continued and the walking got worse, and with countless trips to the doctor's office and to the hospital, no one could say what was wrong.

Finally my blood results came back: I had elevated liver functions and my white blood cell count was off-balance, which was an indication that I had a tick borne illness called Ehrlichiosis. I was then put on ten days of doxycycline, a very commonly used antibiotic prescribed to treat Lyme disease and other tick borne diseases. With taking the doxycycline, I started to feel better! Most importantly, my walking improved.

After the ten days were up, I was not 100% better. That's when my pediatrician at the time said it wasn't Lyme, and if it was in fact Lyme, I would 'be healed'. You can imagine what I was diagnosed with next. I then became one of hundreds of people who are misdiagnosed with the 'it's-all-in-your-head' and post viral syndrome diagnoses. Summer vacation was ending, and I was far too sick to attend my junior year of school, or dance lessons. I just wanted to be healed and go back to doing all of the things that I loved.

I went several months before I was treated again. All of the progress that I had made faded, and I quickly declined neurologically. I started using a walker, and then was dragging myself with the walker, then crawling around the house. I finally and fortunately got to Dr. Charles Ray Jones, the most well-known Lyme guru for children and adolescents. I found out that it was not all in my head, nor post viral syndrome. I had Lyme disease, and previously Lyme meningitis. With blood results, I came back positive with the following: Babesia Microti, Babesia Duncani, Ehrlichiosis, Rocky Mountain spotted fever, Chlamydophila Pneumoniae, Mycoplasma Pneumoniae, and EBV.

Soon enough, I was paralyzed from the hips down. The weakness got progressively worse. Every morning I had hoped that I'd be able to walk normally again, so I would try to stand and I would fall. There was a particular morning when I woke up and felt absolutely nothing. I still tried and fell down hard yet felt nothing. Nothing. Part of me died that day. Part of me remained hopeful to try again the next day. Little did I know, I would be trying and failing at this for about a year. I didn't understand why this was happening to me. I felt like I was being punished for something that

I didn't do. I felt like God was punishing me and that He turned his back on me. I searched for reasons why this was happening to me. I was too immature to yet realize the messages God was trying to send to me.

I remember getting my wheelchair. My younger sister would have fun pushing me around the house with it fast. New dents were made in the house, in the walls and door jambs, but that didn't even come close to being equivalent to the dent in my heart. I was stubborn. I went through a period of refusal towards using the wheelchair. I would drag my entire body around the house, under extreme physical pain that the upper half of my body was in. I would do the army crawl up and down the stairs. Then I realized that I had to use the wheelchair. I didn't want to I had no other choice. My doctors weren't too sure on whether I was going to walk again. Nothing was working, and that really frightened me. I would try my very hardest to get my legs to move, but they were dead. I remember my neurologist testing my reflexes, and there were none. I was so afraid that they were right, that I would never walk again but I decided that they were wrong. I WAS going to walk again. It WILL happen and I will make it happen. I was going to prove every doctor wrong that crossed my path that doubted my future hopes of walking again. I knew it was going to be hard, there were going to be good days and bad days, but I was up for the challenge.

I didn't want to be seen by anyone, including my family. I was self-conscious of myself, because I did not look the same. Dark rings descended from my tired, glossy eyes. My hair was falling out and becoming thin. My skin was pale and sickly to its appearance. I didn't want anyone to see me in my wheelchair, because I knew people were looking; their eyes felt like daggers going through me as they glared. I knew that people made fun of others with disabilities, and I didn't want to go through that cruelty. I just wanted to crawl under a rock and pray to God that I would be better. I would go to stores and people wouldn't even hold a door open for me. It was a struggle to get around some stores, which would really frustrate me because it reminded me that I wasn't like the 'normal ones' anymore. I felt like I was living in a completely different world than the normal ones. My social life suffered, which is extremely hard for teenagers. Being sick was lonely, it is painful on many levels. I would give anything up to be healthy again. I learned quickly that in life, the greatest wealth is health' nothing comes above that.

In the midst of the chaos that became my new life, I still continued schooling. I couldn't physically attend, but thankfully my high school supplied me with two fabulous tutors. Dropping out was an option 'just not an option for me. Giving up was not something I wanted to do. I was fighting for my life at this point; there were no ifs, buts, or maybes. I had to continue fighting for the present and future.

Every day I would get up early and get dressed to go to school, even though I was faced with pain in half of my body, fatigue, cognitive issues, and paralysis. People could say I had a very good excuse to not go to school, but I did not use any excuses. I wanted to go to school, and now that I was sick and couldn't physically go, I wish the other students could realize how lucky they were. It was the simple things that now brought me the most joy in life, and school was one of them. It took my mind off of the fact that I was sick, and it gave me something to work towards. If I wanted to go to college and have the career that I wanted, I had to work hard in school, regardless of my hardships. I couldn't read, so my tutors had to read everything to me. My migraines were so bad, but I would work until I was ready to cry. It was extremely difficult to retain all of the information that I learned in the two hours that I spent tutoring a day, so each day my tutors would have to give a brief explanation about what the lessons were about. I studied hard at home as well. It paid off, because each term I made honor roll. This was a huge accomplishment, because of the way Lyme was affecting my cognition.

After school, I went to physical therapy or aquatic therapy. It was upsetting. I could not make a connection to my legs for them to move, but it didn't stop me from trying tirelessly. After therapy, I would go to my neurologist's office. I would pay him a visit almost every day for an IV. The oral antibiotics were failing, and my infections were progressing. I had to get peripheral IVs, because I am at a higher risk of developing blood clots (thanks to a blood clotting factor that I was born with). This was why my IVs would last only a day sometimes not even a day. When it would last a few days, or if I was really lucky, a week, my mom and I would celebrate. I would sit for almost an hour or more, as the nurse would poke me with needles countless times for search of a promising vein that wouldn't collapse or infiltrate. I had bruises up and down my arms, but all of this was in hopes that the IV antibiotics would work.

I was a senior in high school, and I finally got feeling back in my legs. Nine months of hard work and determination got me out of paralysis! I still remember picking my legs up slightly from my wheelchair and wiggling my toes. My legs were so weak and it felt so good to feel again; all old textures became new again. Now I had two goals: to go to prom and to walk to get my diploma. It wasn't easy, especially with surgeries that gave me some setbacks. I wasn't going to let that stop me. I continued my schooling (still making honors), physical and aquatic therapy, and trying anything in my power to get myself to walk. My knees buckled and I had involuntary movements in my legs. My physical therapist had me wear high heels, which got me to stand straight. The spastic, involuntary movements remained. With my five inch heels, I went to prom and walked to get my diploma. Those two moments will be moments that I will remember for the rest of my life; the sense of pride and accomplishment was exhilarating. I felt invincible.

I was accepted to a community college, where I was to pursue my Associates in Science for nursing. This year, I was still in pain, fatigued, had cognitive problems, but I had come too far to quit. I could not walk for very long in my high heels, so I remained in my wheelchair for a majority of the time. I learned through a nerve conduction test that I had two forms of neuropathy: CIDP and small nerve fiber neuropathy. I learned that I had POTS, a form of dysautonomia. I also learned that attributing to my neuropathy causing my leg movements was a disorder called PANDAS. My strep titers were high and my body was producing too many antineuronal antibodies. My body was suffering autoimmune chaos. I was tired of people looking at me when I was standing with my leg movements. People would come up to me and say inappropriate things like, 'You must be excited, you're dancing!' I remember holding back tears when people would make comments on my leg movements. I could not control it and it would make me feel terrible about myself. No matter what life threw at me, I was so hopeful.

All in all, with time I began walking without any aids on Mother's Day weekend. It was the best Mother's Day gift I could have ever given my mother. I screamed and cried tears of joy, as I put one foot in front of the other. I felt like I was in a dream. The only thing that was letting me know it was reality was the physical pain. It was not a normal walk; I could only walk on the balls of my feel and when I stood still, the leg movements were still there. I didn't care, though. This was huge progress! I called my family members to tell them about my good news. I couldn't wait to show my family and the world myself walking. My prayers were answered and my hard work paid off. I felt the cool hardwood floor on my feet, I felt the carpet, and I got to walk in all my flat shoes that I had never worn before. I got to see myself standing in the mirror, modeling my outfit and look at myself at my actual height. I thought it was the coolest thing ever. I felt like a model walking down a runway; it was simply amazing and the most rewarding moment of my life.

The messages that God was sending me are simple. Lyme disease has robbed me of many things and aspects of my life, like my health, my ability to walk, my social life, time I will never get back, and much more. In hindsight, I thought I had been robbed and cheated in life, and that God was punishing me, but actually I am quite blessed. I see life differently than others do, and I have developed a deeper meaning of life. I am so appreciative of the little things in life, especially walking. Walking is now my favorite thing to do. Each day I wake up still amazed that I can still walk. Nothing could ever compare to that; something so little now means the world to me, because I have lived a period in my life without it. When you almost lose your life to a life-altering illness, you learn to never take anything for granted, because when it's gone, you don't know how much you'd give up to get it back.

I am an absolute believer that though I am sick, the universe has big plans for me. Lyme disease has taught me even more to never give up on my goals or dreams. I may be in chronic pain, but I love going to school and I can't wait to be able to work. I am currently going to school to become a nurse and will then further my education to become a nurse of anesthesia. I also want to become an EMT and eventually a firefighter. This illness has given me a bigger purpose in life: to save others' lives and to help others. I am still alive because I am here for a reason, and that reason is to save another's life and get people healthy again so they can live a beautifully blessed, healthy life.

I want to share my advice with other people fighting Lyme disease (Lymies):

1. *Never, never, never give up:* My first appointment with my LLMD, I saw a plaque which read the words, 'Never, never, never give up!' From that moment on, those words have been in my mind, body, and soul throughout my battle. Lyme is TOUGH; however, you are tougher. Whether you need to speak these words to yourself, or put them in a place where you can be reminded of them and their meaning often, do so. You WILL overcome the war.

2. *Set goals for yourself (big and small!):* I have found that with battling Lyme disease, it is vital to set goals. It's a healthy form of healing. Start out with small goals, for example, getting out of bed for a few minutes or try to make it to that family party. Also set long-term goals. A big one for me was to walk again. It's important for us Lymies to still feel like we are working for something, and accomplishing these goals can give ourselves a sense of pride and self-worth. Know that you can accomplish anything through hard work and keeping your eyes on the prize.

3. *Celebrate all of your victories (no matter how small!):* Celebrate the times you got out of bed for a few hours or for going for a walk. These are great things you are doing! You are pushing through day by day with one of the most misunderstood illnesses in the world. Why not give yourself a pat-on-the-back and celebrate? Watch your favorite movie, indulge in a yummy snack you deserve it!

4. *Take a step back and look at where you once were in your battle:* I think all Lymies are superheroes. We are so strong, but we all have these bad days where we want to throw in our capes and call it quits. When I have these days, I step back and remind myself where I was four years ago. I look at pictures of hospital stays and tests I've gone through, and I realize it's not the end. If it wasn't the end four years ago, it isn't the end now. So take a day to yourself, but remember that the superhero cape only comes off on laundry days!

5. *Be blessed:* You are a miracle! Do you realize that? (I hope so!) You are so blessed! Be blessed for the basic things: family and friends that have stuck by your side during your illness, your spouse or significant other, for your pets, for still being alive. Be blessed for the little things: coffee, your favorite gluten-free treat, your amazing LLMD. There is a lot to still be blessed for! I am blessed to be alive and to be walking. I am not healthy, but I am not dead and that is huge. Do not lose sight of these things throughout the course of your battle.

6. *Uncover your purpose: The higher power and universe has big plans for you. You were given your hardships for the greater good. Maybe you have uncovered your newfound purpose, or maybe it has not found you yet (if you haven't found it yet, be patient!). Once you have found your purpose, put it to use! If you want to go and be an advocate for Lyme, set up a support group in your community. Fulfill your purpose and do it with heart. You will be making a difference in our world. Something positive is going to come out of something negative.*

7. *Learn from your illness: Life is filled with lessons to learn, but pay close attention to the ones you learn with Lyme. Be like a sponge and absorb them all: these are lessons that not many people who are healthy will quite understand, and are lessons that you will carry with you for the rest of your life. My biggest lesson is to appreciate the little things that life has to offer; I still love feeling new textures on my feet since regaining feeling in my legs and walking! With learning these lessons, don't forget to practice them in your everyday life!*

8. *Laugh it out: Keep your sense of humor! When I got my walker, I named it 'Texas Ranger' (Get it?). Laughing is the best medicine around, and has so many benefits: it releases endorphins (our feel-good chemicals), it helps boost the immune system, it's great for stress relief, it relaxes the body, and plus, who doesn't love a good belly laugh?*

9. *Keep your faith close to you: Never give up on God (or whoever it is that you believe in). They say to lay all of your troubles at the Lord's feet and he will take care of them. This is true. It may not be immediate, but have trust in Him. Your faith will give you strength on days where you are weak, clarity on days where you are uncertain, and hope on days where you are discouraged.*

10. *Have patience: Patience is a virtue! Patience is difficult to have, especially when you are sick and all you want is*

relief from your illness. Know that you will get there! Your persistence and hard work will pay off. The climb up this mountain is difficult; there will be setbacks and events that will test your patience. When you get to the top of the mountain, you will love the view. You will see that everything that you have done during this climb was well worth it, because you have your health back.

I don't want people to just learn about the astronomical effects of Lyme disease through my story. I want them to learn something much deeper than that: I want them to appreciate life. I want them to love themselves. I want them to follow their dreams and accomplish their goals. I want them to fight for a better life. I want them to know that if it be Lyme, an illness, or a different hardship, that they can overcome it. After every storm comes sunshine. Find promise in that. I might have had a blueprint of my life when I was sixteen, but life doesn't always go according to plan. My life has not gone the way I expected it, but I am incredibly fortunate'I wouldn't change my life for anything, because I have taken so many positive lessons out of my illness and have matured greatly from it. I will continue to work hard at everything that I aspire to do in life, especially conquering Lyme disease. Life doesn't end; it simply just goes on to the next chapter. Lyme disease is just a chapter in my life. I may not be able to tell the future, but I know how this chapter of my life will end: I will have a happily healthy after. I will get my happily healthy after, and so will you.'

Marissa Cassella

Mindset to Achieve Outstanding Health

66The truth of the matter is that there's nothing you can't accomplish if: (1) You clearly decide what it is that you're absolutely committed to achieving, (2) You're willing to take massive action, (3) You notice what's working or not, and (4) You continue to change your approach until you achieve what you want, using whatever life gives you along the way. 99

Anthony Robbins

After interviewing Lyme survivors, I can reassure you that their mindset was much more important than their financial situation, family support, or even state of their immune system to begin with or level of their illness. And my goal is to teach you how to create that same mindset that will lead to outstanding health.

First off, ask yourself *why* is it an absolute MUST to get your health back. You have to clearly define your *why*, your reason. For some of you it may be your kids or your loved one. You may want to have more energy to be able to enjoy your family. For some of you it may be a particular goal that you are going to achieve as soon as you get your health back. For me it was an ABSOLUTE MUST to reclaim my health and my life - whatever it took. And the reason was because I would never settle for that low of a quality of life. I knew I had so much potential and I was hungry enough to get the breakthrough. But my main drive was not just about myself. After I got sick and was going through a living hell, I told myself I have to get better no matter what to help others with Lyme. Like everybody else I was asking myself *"Why me?"* when I first became sick. And my only answer was – because I HAVE TO FIND A WAY TO RECOVER in order to help others.

After you know why you MUST get your health back, it's time to get into a state of *absolute certainty* that you are winning this battle WHATEVER IT TAKES! Because only a state of *absolute certainty* will make you take *massive actions*. And what action you take will define which results you get. For example John and Maya both have the same symptoms today – extreme fatigue, brain fog, headache, and depression. John whines and complains that he is sick. He takes a bag of chips and a pint of ice cream and plops down on a couch to watch TV. Maya, on the other hand, asks herself: *"What can I do right now to ease my symptoms?"* Maya makes fresh squeezed veggie juice and goes for hot yoga. She is not able to do it full strength, but she does what she can – stretches, practices pranayama (yogic breathing), and meditates. Results: Next morning John is even sicker and more depressed. Maya feels so much better even the same evening. Her brain fog subsided, she is not depressed anymore because she knows her condition is temporary and she is getting better day by day. Good news for Maya; (for John it's actually bad news) the result is *cumulative*. In a few months Maya is feeling so much better and she is *absolutely certain* she is capable of overcoming her health "opportunity", while John lost all his hope; he is feeling worse and worse and acquiring even more destructive habits and behaviors.

In order to be able to push yourself to do something uncomfortable, you need to produce desirable results in your head. Envision yourself being healthy again, even healthier than pre-disease! Imagine what you can do with all that energy! Trust me, if you imprint this in your mind – your body will follow! Because we all have the potential to achieve enormous results but not all of us do. Why? Let me give you an example. For years, so many athletes had tried and failed to run a mile in less than four minutes that people made it out to be a physical impossibility. The world record for a mile was 4 minutes and 1.3 seconds, set by Gunder Hagg of Sweden in 1945. Because of the psychological mystique surrounding the four-minute barrier, no one was able to beat it. In Oxford, England, 25-year-old medical student Roger Bannister cracks track and field's most notorious barrier: the four-minute mile. Bannister, who was running for the Amateur Athletic Association against his alma mater, Oxford University, won the mile race with a time of 3 minutes and 59.4 seconds. First off, as Roger explains, he had to produce results in his mind in order to create a state of certainty. When he was 100% confident in his mind he was able to break the record, his body just followed. Did he have the potential before that? Yes. But his mindset produced the results first. Guess what happened next? All of the sudden to run a mile in less than four minutes became *possible,* and in the next two years 37 athletes broke the record! Believe it's possible and your body will follow!

As Tony Robbins says, *"Change your state and you change your life."* And yes, it does apply to all of us, healthy and not so healthy *yet.* You can change your state in a heartbeat in so many ways and they are all so simple.

The problem is that so many people are looking for the most comfortable ways to change their state without even being aware of it most of the time. People tend to overeat, munch on sugar, drink alcohol, smoke, or take a drug – like a painkiller, none of which addresses the root of the problem. It's only a Band-Aid. And unfortunately all of those "Band-Aids" have tragic consequences, which are cumulative, so most of us don't even see the danger until it's too late. That's what happened to Michael Jackson, Elvis Presley and so many other people, and keeps happening to many more people every single day. It's like a frog in a kettle being slowly simmered to death. If the frog had been dropped into a full boiling pot, the shock of the heat would have caused him to jump back out immediately – but with the heat slowly building up, the frog never notices he is in danger until it's too late to get out.

Since movement can instantly change how we feel, it makes sense for us to create lots of ways to change our state. My favorites are rebounding on my mini trampoline, jogging, hot yoga or sauna and contrast showers (more on that in Part 2). Take a few minutes right now to create *your* ways to change your state. Make a list!

The moment you decide, *"Enough!"* - *"No more"* - *"Sick and tired of being sick and tired,"* and start taking massive actions, your destiny will change! You know 99% of the world's money is being made by 1% of people, because they have conditioned their body and mind and took massive actions. Massive actions produce results... while the rest of the people tell a story of why it did not work and why it is not their fault. Same applies in all areas of our lives, especially in the most important one – health. People that recover from Lyme, cancer, all kinds of autoimmune disorders are not lucky. They do not create a story as to why they are sick and why it is not their fault. You can blame whoever you want – your doctor, your government, your insurance company, your neighbor, your luck; blame will not heal you. *Absolute certainty* in your recovery and *taking massive actions* will!

I have heard a million times from people – *"I am skeptical about this herb/drug/treatment. It is not FDA approved. I have never heard of this before. How come my doctor did not recommend it if it works? Doctors have to prove it to me."* Etc. You get the picture.

No, my friend, you are not skeptical, you are *gutless*! It takes no guts to be skeptical. You don't have to have any capacity to be a critic. It takes guts to *believe*. So the idea, *"they have to prove it to me"* is the biggest lie. This is your fear talking. You are so scared to move out of your comfort zone, scared to be disappointed, scared to fail, that you do not even want to get your hopes up.

And last but not least, I would like to add that we all are defined by our rituals. Let's get back to the example of John and Maya. John wakes up tired and achy which makes him very depressed and hopeless. John pops a few *Tylenols* to cover his aches, then he pops his *Xanax* to make him "happy" and after that he swallows a standard American breakfast: eggs with cheese and bacon, some hash browns, and washes it all down with coffee. Remember, the result is cumulative! John's health deteriorates; he takes more drugs to cover his symptoms and becomes more depressed. Maya wakes up tired and achy as well, but she knows it's temporary; she is going to beat this beast! Maya drinks a glass of water, and then she meditates and then after that goes for a light jog. Her body loosens up due to movement and her aches go away naturally. For breakfast Maya makes herself fresh squeezed green veggie juice and has a bowl of fruit salad. Results – Maya is getting better and better. A year later Maya is vibrant, energetic and fully recovered from her degenerative condition, while John is severely depressed and has developed more health problems. My personal morning ritual is: a glass of water with lemon, rebounding for 10 minutes, dry skin brushing, contrast shower (alternate hot and cold) and then a light breakfast of organic fresh made green veggie juice and a salad. Results – I assisted my body to overcome an "incurable" disease. I feel great, full of energy and excitement!

To achieve anything in life you have to have an absolute faith that you are capable of it. Produce results in your head and take massive actions. And I am here to help. Follow the Master Principles of Vibrant Health in Part 2 as if your life depends on it (and it does!) and you will become the next health billionaire!

Part 2

Master Principles
of Vibrant Health

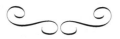

Your Immune System is Your Best Doctor!

66By cleansing your body on a regular basis and eliminating as many toxins as possible from your environment, your body can begin to heal itself, prevent disease, and become stronger and more resilient than you ever dreamed possible! 99

Dr. Edward

I encourage YOU to implement all of these steps into YOUR life – YOU will live the life that you have only dreamed is possible:

An amazingly...

HEALTHFUL

VIBRANT

TRUTHFUL

JOYOUS, and

LOVING LIFE!

Lyme disease is one of the most complicated diseases to treat. While the infections are a significant part of the disease, but impaired physiology, biotoxin load, immune dysfunction, heavy metals, mold, parasites, and psychological break down are what determine how sick a person will be.

There are so many people who get bitten by ticks multiple times and never get sick. There are people that live in highly epidemic areas like Connecticut and New Jersey, and never get sick, and there are people like you and me, that live in Manhattan or other urban areas, and get seriously ill.

There are also people that carry Lyme bacteria, and a whole bouquet of co-infections and viruses and don't have symptoms until a decade later when something happens; commonly six months before they get symptoms. It's usually some kind of trauma, like a car accident, loss of a family member, divorce, loss of a job, break-up or something else. For me it was a break-up; a loss of a guy I was in love with. I remember it as though it happened yesterday. On April 29, 2009 he left the United States for good and we knew we would never be together again. And for the first time in my life I was feeling extremely weak. My body was stiff and in pain due to psychological stress. However, those symptoms went away in a few days and I was back to my normal self. Exactly six months later, October 29, 2009 I woke up with Bell's palsy and was extremely sick. So who knows when I was bitten and for how long I had bugs dormant in my body since I have never had a rash.

The point is that your immune system defines if you are ever going to get sick, how sick you currently are, and how soon you will recover. In this part of the book I will provide you with crucial immune boosting life style changes and treatments that I learned from the best doctors, healers, and survivors all over the world. This new lifestyle saved my life as it has for the lives of thousands before me. All of these treatments are not some kind of "new discovered secret African magic overnight cure". These treatments and lifestyle changes are as old as 5,000 years and proven by generations to be crucial to our health.

These lifestyle changes are an absolute MUST in order to reverse your degenerative illness and obtain your optimum health. Herbs, supplements and treatments are the essential part of healing but are not completely required to get well. *"In order to facilitate the body's ability to heal, those with Lyme must do everything possible to strengthen their immune system. Getting one's health back is a full-time job. The chronically ill need to become aware of how everything affects their health, including their environment, diet, habits, and attitude."* Dr. Ginger Savely, DNP

I agree with what Dr. Paavo Airola has to say about disease and one's immune system: *"Unbelievable as it may seem, the twentieth century concept of disease is not much different from the primitive voodoo concept. The only difference is that the 'evil spirits' have been replaced with 'evil germs', bacteria or virus, which attack the unfortunate and undeserving man… The biological concept of medicine is based on the irrefutable physiological fact that the primary cause of diseases is not the bacteria or virus but the weakened resistance brought about by man's health-destroying living habits and physical and emotional stresses. The bacteria enter the picture only in its final stage."*

Dr. Horowitz defines Lyme disease, Chronic Fatigue Syndrome, Fibromyalgia, and other "mysterious" illnesses as MCIDS, which stands for Multiple Chronic Infectious Disease Syndrome. *"MCIDS would better define patients with chronic borrelia and co-infections, who suffer with chronic fatigue, muscle and joint pain, neuropathy, and neuropsychiatric abnormalities. These patients have multiple overlapping etiologies responsible for their symptoms."* Dr. Horowitz

Antoine Bechamp, a contemporary of Louis Pasteur, said that when it comes to healing the body, the microorganisms are nothing, and the body's environment, or terrain, is everything.

"Obviously, getting enough rest, doing moderate exercise and getting oxygen into cells, taking supplements, doing mild physical therapy and eating well are other lifestyle habits that help the body to heal." Dr. Steven Bock, MD

Dr. Horowitz listed in his presentation the following issues to be treated with Lyme:

1. **Infections:**

a) Bacterial: Lyme disease, Ehrlichiosis, Bartonella, Mycoplasma, Chlamydia, RMSF, Typhus, Tularemia, Q-Fever, Tick paralysis

b) Parasites: Babesiosis and other piroplasms, filiariasis, amebiasis, giardiasis

c) Viruses: EBV, HHV-6, HHV-8, CMV, St Louis Encephalitis, West Nile, Powassan encephalitis and other viral encephalopathies, XMRV virus

d) Candida and other fungi

2. **Immune dysfunction**

3. **Inflammation:** "Sickness syndrome"

4. **Toxicity:** Multiple Chemical Sensitivity, Environmental Illness, Heavy Metals, Mold, and Neurotoxins

5. **Allergies:** foods, drugs, environmental...

6. **Nutritional & Enzyme Deficiencies/** functional medicine abnormalities in biochemical pathways

7. **Mitochondrial dysfunction**

8. **Psychological**

9. **Endocrine disorder**

10. **Sleep disorders**

11. **ANS dys (f)**

12. **G.I.**

13. **Elevated LFT's**

14. **Drug Use/Addiction**

15. **Deconditioning**: Need for PT

As you can see, in order to recover from Lyme (and other degenerative diseases), you have to take care of bacteria, viruses, mycoplasma, parasites, fungi, yeast, mold, heavy metals, neurotoxins, as well as other toxins, food and environmental allergies, nutritional and enzyme deficiencies, psychological, endocrine, and sleep disorders just to name a few.

According to Dr. Paavo Airola, most diseases have the same basic underlying causes. These are: the systematic derangement and biochemical and metabolic disorder brought about by prolonged physical and mental stresses to which the patient has been subjected – such as faulty nutritional patterns, constant overeating, overindulgence in proteins and the body's inability to properly digest them, nutritional deficiencies, sluggish metabolism and consequent retention of toxic metabolic wastes, exogenous poisons from polluted food, water, air and environment, toxic drugs, tobacco and alcohol, lack of sufficient exercise, rest and relaxation, severe emotional and physical stresses, etc. These health-destroying environmental factors bring about derangement in all vital body functions with consequent biochemical imbalance in the tissue, autotoxemia, chronic undersupply of oxygen to the cells, poor digestion and ineffective assimilation of nutrients… *and gradually lowered resistance to disease.* Thus Dr. Airola believes, not the bacteria, but the weakened organism or the lowered resistance is the primary cause of disease. Therefore the only effective way to cure the disease is to eliminate the causes of the diseases. All these underlying causes of ill health, mentioned above, must be corrected before health can be restored.

In the next chapters I will guide you through the necessary changes that will ensure your body will be able to take care of all those problems listed above. As I mentioned in my story, every time I was feeling discouraged, I would read success stories of those who reversed their degenerative diseases. And not just Lyme, but cancer, AIDS, MS, chronic digestion problems, allergies; you name it. And as Tony Robbins says: *"There are patterns of success, people who succeed are not lucky...."* It applies to the biggest success of my life – regaining my health back. I have followed the patterns of those who healed themselves. And I am providing you this pattern that will take you on a road to your best days of health!

You see, about 70% of people have poor health, 20% have good health, a further 8% have excellent health and only 2% have outstanding health. If you are not in this elite 2% then let me tell you it feels incredible and my wish is for you to experience this feeling and way of life, too. It does not matter what your current level of health is, or what age you are. This is possible for you—starting today!

No matter who you are, these principles will work for you. Anyone can practice them, at any age, with any health condition, at any stage of life. Your health does not have to be out of reach, no matter what has happened to you in the past. You can move forward, one step at a time, focus on the next step and just *go*! I did not always think I'd be able to do it. Sometimes I wanted to give up, but I didn't. I always kept moving forward one step at a time. I believe my success in regaining my health is due to that internal drive to say *yes* instead of *no* to life.

The moment you decide that you are 100% committed to getting your health back, no obstacle, no challenge, and no problem will keep you from it. In that moment, your life will change forever and you will be empowered to take control!

Diet Equals Health!

66Let food be your medicine and medicine be your food. 99

Hippocrates

I want you right now to get 100% committed to implementing this most crucial step on your way to recovery. I don't care how many antibiotics, herbs, and supplements you take, chances are very low to recover without changing your diet. Moreover, there are chances of developing some other degenerative diseases such as cancer, leaky gut, IBS, etc., due to an already compromised immune system. Nutrition is the cornerstone and basic foundation for the effective treatment of most conditions including Lyme.

"Modern science has advanced to the point where we have evidence that the right raw materials and nutritional factors can double or triple the protective power of the immune system. If you learn to fill every cell receptor lock with the right nutrient key and meet the demands of each cell, the body's defense takes on super hero qualities – and you will hardly ever get sick again. More important, this change from immunity to Super immunity can save your life." Dr. Joel Fuhrman, MD

When it comes to diet, it is very important to avoid eating "toxins" and "Foods that Kill." These include all kinds of artificial sweeteners, processed sugar, and ALL PROCESSED FOODS, as well as various versions of soy products (90% of soy in the US is genetically modified). *If you can't pronounce it, don't eat it*—Common sense.

To clarify, your diet should be vegan (80% raw), soy-free, sugar-free, casein-free, and wheat-free, consisting of whole organic natural foods. An important part of your diet should be pure water and your diet should contain "Foods That Heal" (super-foods, sprouts), vegetable juices, and fats that heal (omega 3-6-9).

"The most powerful way to heal disease, detoxify and build your body is with vegan food. Stop eating all animals and animal by-products." Dr. Schulze

Over 1.5 million people in America will die **this year alone** because the fat and cholesterol they consumed from eating animals killed them! **That is about 2 people every minute!** There are tons of books and information online about the health-risks of consuming animal products, and there is a tremendous amount of information out there about the healing powers of plant-based foods. The first book that everyone reads and recommends is, *The China Study* by Dr. T. Colin Campbell.

"Meat and dairy consumption must become our diet of the past or we humans have no future! Clearly we can see by our epidemic levels of disease – Diabetes, Heart Disease, Stroke, Obesity, Osteoporosis, etc. – our erroneous meat and dairy consumption is killing us. The simple fact that we have refused to acknowledge is; at this stage of our evolution, we humans are herbivores. Humans are not anatomically or physiologically designed to consume other beings, their secretions (milk) or potential fetuses (eggs) – no matter what our erroneous 'behavioral' beliefs (addictions to fats and sugars) crave.

If your physician has not informed you of this, then there are only two options to consider concerning your physicians competence: either they do not know, or choose not to tell you – not allowed to tell you!? Either way, it is a tragic symptom of our diseased 'health care' system – All the financial incentives are towards sickness." Dr. John McDougall

"We know an enormous amount about the links between nutrition and health. But the real science has been buried beneath a clutter of irrelevant or even harmful information – junk science, fad diets, and food industry propaganda." Dr. T. Colin Campbell, *The China Study*.

"The beef industry has contributed to more American deaths than all the wars of this century, all natural disasters, and all automobile accidents combined. If beef is your idea of `real food for real people,' you'd better live real close to a real good hospital." Neal D. Barnard, M.D., President, Physicians Committee for Responsible Medicine, Washington, D.C

"The human body has no more need for cows' milk than it does for dogs' milk, horses' milk, or giraffes' milk." Dr. Michael Klaper, author of *Vegan Nutrition: Pure and Simple*.

"When we kill the animals to eat them, they end up killing us because their flesh, which contains cholesterol and saturated fat, was never intended for human beings." William C. Roberts, M.D., editor of *The American Journal of Cardiology*

If you feel rebellious and you have all kinds of excuses to continue with your old way of eating, go ahead. But remember, you can't have both- it's either the result or the excuse! *"All truth passes through three stages. First, it is ridiculed. Second, it is violently opposed. Third, it is accepted as being self-evident."* Arthur Schopenhauer

If you are not ready to give up your most life destructive habit – animal products and processed food consumption – you might as well give this book away to someone who is. If however, you have made your decision to be 100% committed to reversing your illness and getting your health back – I welcome you aboard!

Dr. Airola says, at least 75% to 80% of your diet should consist of foods in their natural, raw, uncooked state. Your food should be whole, unprocessed and unrefined, and be organically grown in fertile soil. Your food should be grown without the aid of chemical fertilizers and should contain no residue of toxic insecticides, chemical additives or preservatives.

Dr. Schulze says about a vegan diet, *"This is not about some moral crusade, animal rights, People for the Ethical Treatment of Animals, Greenpeace or The Humane Society issue here. It's a simple life-or-death issue. Statistically, animal food is killing you more than anything else."* If this statement works for you – fine, as long as you stop animal product consumption. For me, personally, simple compassion for animals works. I am not able to eat a little tortured living being. I would hate myself for that. My first reason for being vegan is my love and compassion for animals and then my health comes second. But if you do not really care about other living creatures one bit, as Dr. Schulze mentioned, it is a question of life-or-death, and not just an animal's life, but *your* life or death! The choice is yours, my friend!

Gerson Therapy

66The more you eat, the less flavor; the less you eat, the more flavor. 99

Chinese Proverb

There are many wonderful diet therapies and programs that are all vegan and include plenty of fresh vegetable juices. I would like to talk about the Gerson Therapy since I have been to the Gerson clinic in Tijuana, and I have completed Gerson therapy training.

Dr. Max Gerson developed the Gerson Therapy in the 1930s, initially as a treatment for his own debilitating migraines, and eventually as a treatment for degenerative diseases such as skin tuberculosis, diabetes and most famously, cancer.

The Gerson Therapy is a natural treatment that activates the body's extraordinary ability to heal itself through an organic, vegan diet, raw juices, coffee enemas and natural supplements.

With its whole-body approach to healing, the Gerson Therapy naturally reactivates your body's magnificent ability to heal itself – with no damaging side effects. This powerful, natural treatment boosts the body's own immune system to heal cancer, arthritis, heart disease, allergies, and many other degenerative diseases.

The Gerson Therapy's all-encompassing nature sets it apart from most other treatment methods. The Gerson Therapy effectively treats a wide range of different ailments because it restores the body's incredible ability to heal itself. Rather than treating only the symptoms of a particular disease, the Gerson Therapy treats the causes of most degenerative diseases: toxicity and nutritional deficiency.

An abundance of nutrients from copious amounts of fresh, organic juices are consumed every day, providing your body with a super-dose of enzymes, minerals and nutrients. These substances then break down diseased tissue in the body, while coffee enemas aid in eliminating toxins from the liver.

Throughout our lives our bodies are being filled with a variety of carcinogens and toxic pollutants. These toxins reach us through the air we breathe, the food we eat, the medicines we take and the water we drink. The Gerson Therapy's intensive detoxification regimen eliminates these toxins from the body, so that true healing can begin.

The Gerson Therapy regenerates the body to health, supporting each important metabolic requirement by flooding the body with nutrients from about 15- 20 pounds of organically grown fruits and vegetables daily. Most are used to make fresh raw juice; up to one glass every hour, up to 13 times per day. Raw and cooked solid foods are generously consumed. Oxygenation is usually more than doubled, as oxygen deficiency in the blood contributes to many degenerative diseases. The metabolism is also stimulated through the addition of thyroid, potassium and other supplements, and by avoiding heavy animal fats, excess protein, sodium and other toxins.

Degenerative diseases render the body increasingly unable to excrete waste materials adequately, commonly resulting in liver and kidney failure. The Gerson Therapy uses intensive detoxification to eliminate wastes, regenerate the liver, reactivate the immune system and restore the body's essential defenses – enzyme, mineral and hormone systems. With generous, high-quality nutrition, increased oxygen availability, detoxification, and improved metabolism, the cells – and the body – can regenerate, become healthy and prevent future illness.

Fresh pressed juice from raw foods provides the easiest and most effective way of providing high quality nutrition. By juicing, patients can take in the nutrients and enzymes from nearly 15 pounds of produce every day, in a manner that is easy to digest and absorb.

Every day, a typical patient undergoing Gerson Therapy for cancer consumes up to thirteen glasses of fresh, raw carrot/apple and green-leaf juices. These juices are prepared hourly from fresh, raw, organic fruits and vegetables, using a two-step juicer or a masticating juicer combined with a separate hydraulic press.

Gerson Therapy is a proven method for reversing most degenerative illnesses and restoring the person's health. You do not have to follow the exact Gerson Therapy protocol; however your diet MUST be VEGAN, 80% raw, including plenty of fresh vegetable juices. You can look into Dr. Schulze's program; he has one of the highest success rates in reversing degenerative illnesses. For more information visit https://herbdocblog.com

I highly recommend the book, *The Gerson Therapy: The Proven Nutritional Program for Cancer and Other Illnesses*, by Charlotte Gerson and Morton Walker, D.P.M. to learn more about this miraculous therapy.

Since my full recovery I have started a health retreat, called *Health Mastery*, where we practice modified Gerson Therapy, including juice fast, vegan diet, coffee enemas, energy treatments, acupuncture, chiropractic adjustments and sound healing with great success. And the combination of a juice fast and raw vegan diet is the cornerstone of the program. You can read more about the Health Mastery program at http://www.healthmasteryretreat.com

A vegan, organic, gluten-free, casein-free, soy-free, and processed foods–free diet is your ticket to perfect health!

And remember, in any moment a decision you make can change the course of your life forever. I encourage you to make a decision that will cause the positive floodgates to open, and all of the things that you have been waiting for to fall into place.

Body Cleansing

66Garbage in garbage out. 99

George Fuechsel

Detoxification must be an important part of healing. As with many autoimmune cases, there are many factors. Neurotoxin overload can damage both the nervous system and your body's detoxification organs. Exposure to heavy metals, viruses, bacteria, fungi, molds, parasites and protozoans can trigger the overload. Under normal circumstances, your body would excrete toxic substances before they can cause any damage. In the case of neurotoxin overload, exposure limits your body's ability to get rid of the problem, so cumulative exposure can do cumulative damage. Once the nervous system and detoxification organs stop functioning well, accumulating toxins create intracellular damage and greater susceptibility to the effects of disease. It may make the progression of disease in your body faster or more severe.

In the case of Lyme disease, the guilty party is a "smart" bacterium. To protect itself from the immune system, it "hides" inside your body. This causes clogging in your lymphatic system and thickening blood as they neurotoxic Lyme bacteria cower from your natural defenses. Because your blood thickens, it cannot flow as well, and no longer does its job inside your body: the liver's waste disposal mechanisms become sluggish and the interstitial fluid becomes too sticky. This stickiness prevents the fluid from picking up waste and other particles that need processing, and further stops it from bringing nourishment to your cells.

Interstitial fluid carries microorganisms, enzymes, proteins, hormones, and other particles to the lymphatic system for processing. Lyme uses this mechanism, as well as the collagen system, to invade every part of your body. Because all of your organs, glands, tissues, and systems are weighed down by Lyme, you become particularly susceptible to other infections, which are often unseen during the course of treatment.

Lyme patients must practice continual detoxification. In addition to lowering immunity from neurotoxins in general, Lyme bacteria create a neurotoxin as they die, polluting the blood, lymph, liver, and colon. Herxheimer (Herx) reactions, consisting of extreme fatigue, headaches, nausea, tingling, and other flu-like symptoms are a common response to toxic overload. Patients already in treatment for degenerative diseases often find their existing symptoms getting much worse, in addition to the "flu" feeling. Detoxification is a crucial part of recovery.

The body has many ways to eliminate waste. The liver takes care of toxins and hormones, and metabolizes proteins and fats. While the colon removes solid waste (feces) the kidneys and bladder are responsible for liquid waste (urine). Bile in the GI tract excretes hormones, and water-soluble toxins are excreted through urine. Your lungs remove gas toxins from the bloodstream. Your skin removes toxins through sweat, and, when overloaded, you breakout in pimples, pustules, abscesses, or sores.

Now, let's start with body cleansing. Body cleansing is an extremely important part of every prevention and healing program. You may be wondering, *"Are dietary changes you make also a form of cleansing?"* Yes, but most people need more than this, especially when it comes to liver health. Body cleansing is even important for children. Our internal organs can hold a lot of toxins and sometimes, it is impossible to get those toxins out without cleansing. Our liver can contain hundreds of intrahepatic stones. Those stones will block bile flow and affect the status of your health; your digestion. Another problem is parasites. You must learn as much as possible about parasites. And don't forget about dental toxins, as well.

Let's start with a cleansing program. You should do cleansing in this order:

1. Bowel cleanse with parasite cleanse

2. Dental cleanup: dental work may be one cofactor of your disease — amalgam, root canal, nickel crowns, and cavitations (pocket inside jaw bone left after extraction of the wisdom and molar teeth).

3. Kidney cleanse

4. Liver cleanse

Bowel Cleanse

66Keeping your bowel flora healthy is the single-most important thing that you can do for your health! 99

Dr. Bernard Jensen

Bowel movements are the basis of your health. If you don't have at least one bowel movement per day, you are already walking your way toward diseases. There is an epidemic in our society, and it has to do with the gastro-intestinal diseases that we develop within us as a result of the food that we eat: Crohn's, Colitis, Diverticulitis, and other diseases of the intestinal tract. COLON CANCER IS THE SECOND LEADING CANCER KILLER IN THE U.S.!

"Did you know that in one form or another cleansing of the large intestine (bowel or colon) has been practiced since 1500 BC (over 3500 years!)? Colon Lavage was first recorded in the Egyptian document, Ebers Papyrus, which dealt with the practice of medicine." The Ebers papyrus is a roll 20.23 m long and 30 cm high; the text is distributed in 108 columns of 20 to 22 lines each. It contains 877 recipes concerning a great variety of diseases or symptoms. The Ebers Papy-

rus comprises of 110 pages, and is by far the lengthiest of the medical papyri. It is dated c. 1534 B.C. However, one portion of the papyrus suggests a much earlier origin.

In any detoxification, dysfunctional bowels are a sign to start there. Gut Associated Lymphoid Tissue (GALT) comprises 60% of your immune system, and is housed in your intestines, so healthy GI functioning is an important step to recovering your body. Natural supplements, colon hydrotherapy, and colon reflorastation therapy can keep the bowels healthy and functional.

Binding agents, such as fiber or chlorella, allow neurotoxins to be eliminated with waste. Without numerous daily bowel movements, colon hydrotherapy, and these binding agents, the neurotoxins stay in your system. Your colon reabsorbs the toxins if they cannot bind, creating a vicious cycle of toxicity and immune dysfunction.

For patients with diarrhea or IBS, it's often better to start with colon reflorastation therapy. Overactive bowels may be a sign that there are not enough good bacteria in the intestinal tract, and colon reflorastation allows probiotics to work directly on the bowels. Stomach acidity often prevents orally administered probiotics from reaching the lower intestine, leading to a low success rate of 2-5%. Rectal administrations, such as colon reflorastation therapy, allow the bacteria to get where they need to go and grow there. The bacteria are there and flourishing within three days, and can be reapplied as needed.

Let's get straight to business. You do need to clean your colon regularly. I recommend professional hydro colon therapies and coffee enemas. You can read about the importance and benefits of colon therapy online or ask your practitioner. Since you have to do coffee enemas much more often (sometimes multiple times per day) and on your own, let's discuss why and how to do them.

The sigmoid colon allows your body to detect toxicity. It is an s-shaped organ located at the end of the colon, right before the rectum. Your body will reabsorb nutrients from the colon if it can, but most nutrients are reabsorbed before reaching the sigmoid colon. The specialized circulatory system that connects the sigmoid colon and the liver lets you know when toxic excrement has reached the rectum. This circuit, known as the enterohepatic circulation, is what may make you feel sick right before you empty your bowels. Once you eliminate the waste, you stop feeling sick because the toxicity is gone. This circulation means that it is very important to use the restroom as soon as you feel the urge to go, allowing the rectum to remain empty, and preventing constant recirculation of toxicity.

Once the toxins reach the liver, they are mitigated by the liver's work. The direct connection between the liver and sigmoid colon exists so that the toxic particles can go straight to the liver instead of wreaking havoc on the rest of the body. Coffee enemas tap into this connection to send caffeine directly to the liver and trigger quick, powerful detoxification. The caffeine makes the liver increase bile production, allowing it to send processed toxins to the small intestine. Alkaloids in the coffee cause higher levels of glutathione S-transferase, which lets your liver make its detoxification pathways function. It also allows more glutathione to be created, which lets your liver produce the bile it needs to eliminate toxins. When the previously processed toxins are eliminated, the liver can process the backlog of toxins hiding in the rest of your body.

If the enema is performed incorrectly, the coffee may enter regular circulation. Proper administration of the coffee enema will target the liver rather than the body as a whole, allowing the liver to detox quickly and begin working on the buildup of toxins in your organs and tissues.

HOW TO PERFORM A COFFEE ENEMA

To perform a coffee enema, you'll need:

-An enema bag or bucket (ideally one you can see through, should not have any strong odors)

-An old towel

-A large, stainless steel pot (for brewing the coffee)

-Caffeinated, organic, drip grind coffee

-Uncontaminated water (if water is chlorinated, boil for 10 minutes to purify)

Step One- Boil a little more than one quart of the water in a pan, and allow it to boil. While it is boiling, add two tablespoons of coffee (more or less if a different amount has been prescribed). Continue boiling for five minutes. Turn the heat off and allow the pan to rest on the burner. The water should be tepid by the time you use it, test it as you would a baby's bottle. For safety's sake, err on the side of keeping it too cool. **Caution: Do not ever use hot or steaming water for an enema.**

Step Two- Lay the old towel down where you have enough space, and carefully carry your pan to it. Set up an area to perform the enema, making it as relaxing as you'd like. You can bring something to read if you feel it will help you relax.

Step Three- Pour your coffee into the enema bucket. Do not allow coffee grounds into the cup, and do not use a paper filter. It may be helpful to use a filtering container (like a teapot) to filter out the coffee grounds. Clamp the catheter of the enema bag, and place the bag in the sink. Pour the coffee into the bag, and briefly release the clamp to let the air bubbles out of the catheter tube. Close the bag by re-clamping the catheter.

Step Four- Hang the enema bucket from a doorknob

or towel rack; keeping it at the right level will produce a gentle flow to clean the rectum and distal sigmoid colon, not the entire colon. If you allow it to flow too deeply, you will experience the general effects of caffeine, which you may not want.

Step Five- Lie on your back or your right side and insert the enema catheter. (Use coconut oil or any other food grade vegetable oil as a lubricant, make sure to a avoid petroleum). Be gentle as you ease the tube a few inches into the rectum. Unclamp the catheter and let the first half of the coffee flow in. Do not let in more than two cups, and stop at the first sign of discomfort or fullness by clamping off the catheter. Remember, this is a gentle enema, so do not try to use an incline board or a different position to force the enema deeper.

Step Six- If you can, "keep" the enema for 12-15 minutes. If you feel the urge to expel it, follow your instincts. Forcing yourself to retain the enema can do more harm than good. Getting rid of the enema quickly still helps clean the colon and you will have an easier time holding it next time you perform the enema. Once you've clamped the catheter, take the tip off and eliminate waste as needed. Repeat this process with the second ½ quart of coffee after you eliminate once.

Step Seven- Once you are finished, rinse the bag and let it dry.

Other Recommendations:

- Remember that your goal is to hold the enema longer, not going through all the coffee.

- Be sure to keep the enema bag clean by regularly letting boiling water, peroxide, or similar cleaners run through the empty bag.

- If these coffee enemas make you feel wired, cause palpitations or irregular heartbeats, or lead you to experience other caffeine-related sensations, use less coffee. Cutting the amount in half for a little while may help.

- Other reasons for strange reactions are non-organic coffee and impure water. Try organic coffee brewed with chemical-free water.

- If, after a week of daily enemas, you never hear or feel a "squirting" of the gallbladder under your right ribcage, consider raising the "dosage" of coffee by adding more coffee per quart. Try raising the amount of coffee by half a tablespoon per quart of water, but make sure not to ever add more than two tablespoons per cup. If this doesn't help, try raising the number of enemas per session to three.

- Stop performing enemas immediately if you feel any kind of ill effect. Discuss adverse reactions with your doctor.

- Do not use enemas more than once a day without medical supervision or consultation. Most users only administer it a few times per week.

I will tell you right now an important point that is beyond the scope of the benefits of coffee enemas but it is so important that it must be brought to your attention: do you drink coffee or any caffeine and you are easily stimulated from it and that feeling lasts for some time? If you answered yes, your body is doing a very poor job at processing toxins, chemicals or other harmful compounds.

This increases your risk of chemical sensitivity, fibromyalgia, fatigue, cancer, autoimmune disease, hormone imbalances and generalized ill health.

Coffee enemas saved me from excruciating headaches

and debilitating fatigue and brain fog. Try to do a coffee enema when you feel tired, achy, and foggy – you will be surprised how fast your symptoms will be relieved. And this is proof that your symptoms are caused by high toxicity and clogged liver (we will be discussing detoxing therapies and liver cleanses further). Also, as mentioned in a previous chapter, coffee enemas are a major part of Gerson Therapy — the most effective therapy for healing cancer and other degenerative diseases. It is also a major part of our program at a *Health Mastery Retreat.*

Parasite Cleanse

66The best and most efficient pharmacy is within your own system. 99

Robert C. Peale

Hookworms, roundworms, pinworms, lungworms, and liver flukes are only some of the parasites that may live in our organs. They live in our intestinal walls, and in brains, hearts, lungs, and livers, stealing nutrients that our bodies should be using. This "leeching" means that we have fewer nutrients, vitamins, minerals, and other food with which to heal our bodies and function at our best.

You can acquire parasites through contact with almost anything: including the air! One sample of almost 3000 people found that 32% tested positive for some kind of parasitic infection. That number is probably higher when you have a chronic illness: When you're healthy, your body can reject these parasites, but people with limited immune functioning cannot push out parasites the way that healthy bodies do. If you have a chronic illness, especially one that affects your immune system like Lyme your body may become a repository of parasitic activity.

Parasites can leech many of your much-needed fuel, and you wouldn't even know it!

When you have a parasitic infection, your GI tract becomes inflamed, and you can no longer absorb nutrients. Parasites produce acid, making your nervous system sluggish, damaging your organs and breaking down your muscle tissue. Your liver and kidneys also experience sluggishness, because of toxins that parasites produce. This vicious cycle allows more parasites and other problems (like yeast) to take root in your system.

Because parasites can cause so much damage and still go overlooked, many doctors who specialize in Lyme recommend that patients undergo treatment for parasites as well. Dr. Klinghardt suggests that treatment for parasites can be just as important as treatment for Lyme itself. Using a bowel cleanser will help flush out the parasites and the toxins and eggs they've produced, from your system. Most parasites have a 21 day life cycle, so your treatment should last 23+ days.

Dr. Hulda Clark says, *"Getting rid of all parasites would be absolutely impossible using clinical medicines that can kill only one or two parasites each. Such medicines also tend to make you quite ill. Imagine taking 10 such drugs to kill a dozen of your parasites! Good news, perhaps, for the drug makers but not for you.*

Yet three herbs can rid you of over 100 types of parasites! And without so much as a headache! Without nausea! Without any interference with any drug that you are already on! Does this sound too fantastic? Just too good to be true? They are nature's gift to us. The herbs are:

Black Walnut Hulls (from the black walnut tree)

Wormwood (from the Artemisia shrub)

Common Cloves (from the clove tree)

These three herbs must be used together. Black walnut hull and wormwood kill adults and developmental stages of at least 100 parasites. Cloves kill the eggs. Only if you use them together will you rid yourself of parasites. If you kill only the adults, the tiny stages and eggs will soon grow into new adults. If you kill only the eggs, the million stages already loose in your body will soon grow into adults and make more eggs. They must be used together as a single treatment."

It will probably take some time to find a good parasite treatment: fresh Black Walnut is hard to find, and Cloves and Wormwood may vary in potency. While there are many websites that sell this combination of herbs, some of them will work, while others aren't worth your time or money. Learning everything you can about industry standards will help you make informed decisions when buying herbs. The price for a 1 month supply of herbs is anywhere from $14 to $350. I am not here to endorse any product, however I find that the cheaper the product is, the less potent it is and products from the health food stores usually do not work. Please consult your naturopath or read reviews online.

Dental Clean Up

MERCURY AMALGAMS

66The human body has been designed to resist an infinite number of changes and attacks brought about by its environment. The secret of good health lies in successful adjustment to changing stresses on the body. 99

Harry J. Johnson

It is more toxic than lead, cadmium and even arsenic. It is mercury, and it's in your "silver" tooth fillings. Dentists have been using a combination of metals (including mercury) to make these fillings for decades. The fillings are marked as biohazards when they arrive at the dentist's office (it even comes in the biohazard container), and to dispose of it, the office follows hazardous materials protocol. Does that sound safe?

The fillings are called "dental amalgams" and they are made up of mercury (50%), silver (35%), tin (15%) and various other metals. Sweden, Canada, and Germany have imposed serious limitations on the use of mercury in dental amalgams, or banned it all together. The World

Health Organization (WHO) believes that mercury from these fillings can leak into the body, and may be responsible for illnesses such as ME/CFS, multiple sclerosis, Alzheimer's, and many auto-immune diseases. As we know, any damage to the immune system can be disastrous. Another area where dental amalgams wreak havoc is the nervous system, especially during development. Some researchers believe that the increased rates of developmental disorders such as autism may be linked to the use of mercury in vaccines.

Mercury is also implicated in mood disorders. Many mood and developmental disorders are linked to allergic/immune responses, which are triggered by the inhibition of cellular enzymatic processes due to mercury. Immune reactivity tests have uncovered the effects of mercury on autoimmune diseases. In the body, it binds with the hydroxyl radical in amino acids, linking it to disorders such as autism, schizophrenia, lupus, eczema and psoriasis, scleroderma, and allergies.

Why don't dental amalgams use the word mercury instead of "silver"? Mercury is not safe at any level of exposure: small amounts of mercury can damage many major organs and glands, affecting hormone levels and immune function. When pregnant women are exposed to mercury, tiny particles can even change the developing brain inside them. Autopsy studies have found an intense correlation between the number of dental amalgams and the amount of mercury found in the brain.

In patients who had Alzheimer's, researchers found high levels of mercury in the brain. Other examples of mercury's disastrous neurological impacts come from research that relates the effects of mercury to the pathological effects seen in Lou Gehrig's disease (ALS). Spinal fluid from patients with Alzheimer's and ALS demonstrates the ways in which mercury stops natural detoxification of the body through enzyme systems.

In the case of dental amalgams, mercury vapor and abraded particles leak from the fillings. This leakage dramatically increases when people chew, brush, or drink hot liquids. Daily intake of mercury from dental fillings may be higher than the combined intake from air, water, and food (even fish!). You absorb the vapor through inhalation and swallowing. Another source of vapor may be your own body! Because mercury damages your intestinal system, the microorganisms that live there learn how to resist mercury and antibiotics. This means that antibiotic treatment for diseases such as Lyme becomes less effective, and that mercury that ends up in your intestinal tract gets converted into vapor again and taken back up into your body.

The American Dental Association insists that there is no problem with dental amalgams (they claim there is "no evidence" demonstrating that it causes disease). Despite their claims, patients with chronic problems (especially with issues like yeast sensitivity) often find that their problems are greatly reduced by the removal of dental amalgams. People with any kind of immune functions should consider doing the same: why keep them when there is a chance they are hurting your recovery? If you're already weakened by the disease, there is no need to add additional barriers to recovery.

In fact, the symptoms of Lyme disease and mercury poisoning overlap quite a bit. You may be suffering from one or both of them without knowing which combination you have. Removing your fillings can be an excellent first step towards reducing symptoms and determining the cause.

Find a biological dentist in your area who can safely

remove mercury amalgams from your mouth. *"Biological dentistry combines the techniques and artistry of general dentistry with a focus on the implications oral health has on the entire body. Biological dentistry recognizes the link between oral health and general health. A biological dentist appreciates that the diseases and materials in your mouth can have lasting, negative effects on other systems in your body. Biological dentists also work with other like-minded health care providers to assess the compatibility of dental materials, to provide nutritional support, and, if needed, to provide detoxification from the damaging effects of oral toxins. The biological dentist keeps your whole health in mind, not just the condition of your teeth and mouth."*

REAL CASE:

CHRONIC FATIGUE SYNDROME

By the time he came to acupuncturist M.M. Van Benschoten, O.M.D., practicing in Reseda, California, Albert, age 37, had been beset by chronic fatigue syndrome for 7 years. He reported headaches, chest pain, fatigue, lymph node swelling, muscle aches, irritability, and light-headedness.

Although Albert had elevated blood levels of Epstein-Barr virus, normally associated with chronic fatigue, Dr. Van Benschoten's analysis of Albert's acupuncture meridians (energy pathways through the body) showed no indication of bacterial or viral activity capable of producing his symptoms.

Instead, he found mercury toxicity from dental amalgams to be the fundamental underlying cause of the suppression of Albert's immune system.

To arrive at this conclusion, Dr. Van Benschoten used an energy medicine device in an analytical approach called, "acupoint biophoton diagnostics."

Toxic metals such as mercury interfere with the normal en-

ergy patterns in various acupuncture channels; harmful energies set up interference patterns ("biophoton" emissions) in the meridians, in this case, the heart channel, explains Dr. Van Benschoten.

He prescribed a series of Chinese herbs, including chrysanthemum, angelica dahurica, isatis, bupleurum, cnidium, astragalus, salvia, platycodon, siler, taraxacum, ligustrum lucidum, and fructus lycium. After taking these herbs for 6 weeks, Albert was headache-free and had relief from fatigue and chest pain.

The degree to which mercury toxicity was interfering with his energy pathways also was reduced.

Three months later, Albert had 14 mercury amalgams removed.

However, on his next visit, Dr. Van Benschoten found that the mercury interference had increased. 'Over-zealous removal of all amalgam fillings can significantly increase the patient's mercury levels if done without adequate precautions during amalgam removal and proper mercury detoxification therapy,' notes Dr. Van Benschoten.

He instructs his patients to wear an oxygen mask during amalgam removal, in addition to having their dentists use a rubber dam and high speed suction with water.

But Dr. Van Benschoten says that Chinese herbal medicines successfully help detoxify the patient and restore immune function after mercury amalgam removal.

He prescribed a second series of herbs, including moutan, taraxacum, prunella, glycyrrhiza, grifola, ligustrum lucidum, and verbena to clear the mercury from Albert's system.

After taking them for several months, Albert reported he was still free from chronic fatigue and that he had a stronger resistance to infection.

Danger of Root Canals, Cavitations

Where is the evidence? The American Dental Association (ADA) claims that root canals are completely safe, but they have published no evidence to support that claim. After a root canal, teeth may become incubators for deadly bacteria, which can enter your blood stream under certain conditions. Many scientists have warned against the dangers of root canals for over a century, but ignorant dentists insist it is totally safe. Dentists perform 41,000 root canals every day in the U.S. alone. Patients who believe they are undergoing a perfectly routine and safe procedure may be setting themselves up for disaster.

Your root-canalled teeth may contain toxic anaerobic bacteria. When these bacteria are released into your bloodstream, it can cause many serious medical conditions. The effects may not show up right away, some don't manifest for decades, but once they do, they can be deadly. After the procedure, the risk remains in place for many years. Because the disease doesn't happen right away, doctors and patients may have trouble tracing the "root" cause of the disease destroying your system.

Your teeth provide the perfect incubator for deadly bacteria. They are made up of a soft internal chamber, a hard mineral mid-layer, and finally, the white part that you can see as an outer case. They are held in your mouth by connections made of "periodontal ligament" and dentists learn that there are one to four major canals per tooth. They don't even learn about the 3 miles of accessory canals that, like branching blood vessels, also aid your teeth. These canals aid the movement of microorganisms which is useful while your teeth are alive. Weston Price (westonaprice.org) has identified 75 separate canals in a single tooth. Hal Huggins, DDS, MS, provides supporting evidence on westonaprice.org. After a root canal, these accessory canals are still open, but none of the support systems that prevent the growth of bad bacteria are still in place, allowing toxic anaerobic bacteria to flourish.

During the procedure, the tooth is hollowed out then filled with gutta-percha, a substance that cuts it off from its support system. When the bacteria are cut off from support systems such as blood, they remain hidden in your teeth, separated from treatments like antibiotics and the natural defenses of the body. Because they are no longer a part of your body's natural systems, the good bacteria grow into their new, toxic form. They are antibiotic resistant because they are hidden from the body, and harder to destroy because they are stronger. They wait in your teeth and, if they are ever reintroduced to your body, they can be very destructive.

Attempts to neutralize this threat have proven ineffective because the tooth is such a great hiding place. Nearly every root-canalled tooth contains these bacteria, but it cannot be reached by conventional methods like antibiotics. An infection by these bacteria can cause immediate and serious damage as soon as it enters your jaw. It begins by forming "cavitations" pockets of dead tissue in your jawbone. These cavitations are followed by infection and gangrene. They are a known risk of tooth extraction (like having your wisdom teeth removed), but have also been found after root canals.

Your body has trouble identifying and healing cavitations. The Weston Price Foundation found only two out of 5,000 surgeries in which cavitations had healed themselves. The initial infection also has few symptoms; so many root-canal patients may have this problem without knowing it! When the bacteria migrate from the cavitations to your bloodstream, they can nest in your organs, glands, and tissues causing heart, kidney, rheumatic, neurological and autoimmune diseases. They may even cause cancer.

Dr. Price implanted fragmented root-canalled teeth of humans who had experienced heart attacks into rabbits, and found that the rabbits died of heart disease within a few weeks. This method transferred the heart diseases of humans to the rabbits every time, and other diseases 80% of the time. Dr. Robert Jones surveyed 300 cases of breast cancer, and found that 93% of breast cancer patients had had a root canal, and the rest had other kinds of oral pathologies. In most of the cases he looked at, the tumor developed on the same side of the body as the root canal. His findings are supported by Dr. Josef Issels, who has worked with cancer patients for 40 years and found that 97% of his patients had root canals. Dr. Jones believes that the toxic bacteria inhibit the proteins that normally prevent tumors from developing in the body.

When your immune system is compromised, these bacteria can spread unchecked. One study found that about 400% more bacteria lived in the area around the root-canaled tooth than the tooth itself. Even more bacteria lived in the bone around the teeth. This finding implies that the tooth functions as an incubator and eats the bone in your jaw causing cavitations. When you have Lyme or another disease that damages your immune system, stopping the spread of these vicious bacteria can become extremely difficult.

The root canal is a dangerous procedure, and the only medical procedure in which a dead body part is left to fester in the body. Your body has natural mechanisms for removing medical waste, but these do not apply to teeth that are removed from the blood supply, and a weakened immune system can make this situation even worse.

Your immune system doesn't care for dead substances, and just the presence of dead tissue can cause your system to launch an attack, which is another reason to avoid root canals — they leave behind a dead tooth.

I strongly recommend never getting a root canal. Risking your health to preserve a tooth simply doesn't make sense. Unfortunately, there are many people who've already had one. If you have, you should seriously consider having the tooth removed, even if it looks and feels fine. Remember, as soon as your immune system is compromised, your risk of developing a serious medical problem increases — and assaults on your immune system are far too frequent in today's world.

I strongly recommend consulting a biological dentist because they are uniquely trained to do these extractions properly and safely, as well as being adept at removing mercury fillings, if necessary. Their approach to dental care is far more holistic and considers the impact on your entire body — not JUST your mouth.

If you need to find a biological dentist in your area, I recommend visiting toxicteeth.org, a resource sponsored by Consumers for Dental Choice. This organization, championed by Charlie Brown, is a highly reputable organization that has fought to protect and educate consumers so that they can make better-informed decisions about their dental care. The organization also heads up the Campaign for Mercury-Free Dentistry.

I found one of the best biological dentists in Tijuana, Mexico: Dr. Solorio. I am so grateful to Dr. Solorio for the amazing job he has done and for the amazing care he took of me.

Kidney Cleanse

If you're experiencing: unexplained lower back pain, an inability to rid yourself of excess water weight, kidney stones, or a urinary tract infection, you may want to try a kidney cleanse. Cleansing your kidneys lets them detox and rest so that they can begin working well, improving the overall health of your immune system, detoxification systems, and your body.

Kidney cleanses improve health by flushing out toxins and dissolving kidney stones made of accumulated, difficult to process debris. Different salts build up inside your kidney, and eventually become crystals in your urine. When these crystals become large enough, they are called kidney stones. Stones come in a variety of types: some take days to dissolve, while others require months; some can be dissolved with water, while others require more targeted combinations of palliatives. The urethra and bladder can also contain stones. These stones are made up of minerals and other chemicals that may come from your diet.

Conditions such as dehydration or infection can encourage the formation of crystals. Dehydration reduces the amount of urine and infection increases the amount of salts that tend to become crystals. Both processes lead to a higher amount of salt than urine, which stops the salt from dissolving, encouraging the formation of kidney stones.

Cleansing your kidneys requires a lot of clean water that does not contain the chemicals found in public water supplies. To properly function, your kidneys require the consumption of half of your body weight in clean water every day. Juice fasting and eating only raw fruits and vegetables can also help take the burden off of your kidney so that it can rest and detox. Watermelon is a particularly useful kidney support fruit (if you juice it, be sure to include the rind). Foods high in vitamin C and vitamin B6 can also be extremely helpful (consider taking supplements containing these vitamins to be sure you're giving your kidney all the support it needs). Other helpful foods include cranberries, parsley, aloe vera, wheatgrass, cucumber, celery, juniper berries, marshmallow root, ginger root, wild carrot, and uva ursi (with care).

10 STEPS TO CLEANSE YOUR KIDNEYS:

Step One- Water: You should be drinking half your weight in water every day. During the cleanse, drink 3 quarts of water per day. Make sure this water is clean through filtering or other purification methods: the point of this cleanse is to give your kidneys a break! Fresh spring water is recommended to prevent your kidneys from accumulating acid and other waste. As you already know, consuming a sufficient amount of water is crucial in any detoxification process.

Step Two- No Soda: The sugar and caffeine in soft drinks dehydrates your body, and the sugar also stimulates the release of insulin, which puts additional strain on your heart. A crucial step in cutting out processed foods is cutting out soft drinks. I hope you have already quit all sugars and processed foods by now!

Step Three- No Caffeine or Alcohol: when you drink beer or coffee, your body gets rid of three times what you drink in water. As diuretics, they can cause perpetual dehydration when consumed routinely. Giving up these drinks can keep your kidneys healthy by making sure your body has enough water. It is especially crucial for chronically ill people with weakened immune systems.

Step Four- Lemon Juice: Combine the juice from one lemon with clean, warm water and drink it every morning. This will aid both your kidneys and your liver.

Step Five- Sweat: The more you sweat, the more your body has a chance to get rid of toxins that must otherwise go through your lungs, colon, and kidneys.

Step Six- No Red Meat: Consuming animal protein, especially the kind found in red meat, can produce uric acid which leads to kidney stones. If your kidneys are overwhelmed, they can't get rid of the acid and your body stores it as gout crystals in parts of your body with bad circulation.

Step Seven- More Green Food: Eating or drinking greens helps alkalize the body, preventing acid waste from building up. Meat, cheese, and processed foods raise the amount of acid waste in your body.

Step Eight- Exercise Vigorously: Exercising vigorously for 20 minutes daily activates the lymph system, which allows your kidneys to take a break. Activating multiple systems each day can help distribute toxin processing and stop one system from getting overburdened.

Step Nine- Stop Using Drugstore Painkillers: Any drug you consume goes through your liver and kidneys. Over the counter painkillers fatigue both systems, preventing your body from processing other waste.

Step Ten- Use Special Kidney Cleansing Herbs on a regular daily basis to help cleanse, repair and maintain peak kidney function for life. (I recommend Dr. Schulze's and H. Clark's Kidney Cleanse Teas)

While writing this chapter, I came across the following recent blog post on Dr. Schulze's website. I really want to share it with you, my friends, to prove how powerful kidney cleansing is!

"Dear Dr. Schulze,

My daughter is 9 now; one year ago she was told that she had a tumor in her bladder. It was found in an ultrasound and the photo was there to prove it. She had had many UTI's (Urinary Tract Infections) and even a recent kidney infection. We were told to go to Seattle Children's Hospital and the appointment was 4 weeks away. The first thing we did was put her on your 5 Day Kidney cleanse. My husband and I had done cleanses before, but never our children. At 8 years old with this huge scare, we talked her into doing the cleanse. She was AMAZING! She zipped through your cleanse way better than my husband and I did! We could not believe it! She would take her shot of Detox formula with some white grape juice and say, 'What's the big deal?!'

(4 weeks later at the Seattle Children's Hospital) Well, guess what, after an extensive test, the polyp/growth/tumor... WAS GONE!

The doctor showed it to me on the ultrasound disc I brought to her, but it was no longer there! I was told to go home and be thankful! I got into my rental car and cried with relief!"

Liver/Gallbladder Cleanse, Flush

Stress, environmental toxins, processed and fried foods all lead to liver dysfunction. Forcing the liver to process everything we deal with in the modern world can overburden it, which stops it from processing toxins and fats effectively. Eating foods known to help the liver alleviates this stress, letting your body clean itself once again. To further aid your liver, take a liver-cleansing supplement and do at least two liver and gallbladder cleanses every year. Try to maintain the liver-cleansing diet in your daily life to keep your liver working well.

THE LIVER CLEANSING DIET:

Spices and Teas: Whole **garlic** naturally contains high amounts of allicin and selenium which are known to help the liver. It activates liver enzymes which are crucial for flushing out toxins. **Turmeric** helps enzymes get rid of carcinogens (and is easy to add to most veggie dishes.) **Green Tea** is famously full of antioxidants that promote healthy liver function.

Fruits: **Grapefruit** contains vitamin C and other antioxidants that help the liver process toxins. Drinking a small glass of grapefruit juice boosts production of detoxification enzymes, pushing out toxins and carcinogens. **Lemons and Limes** also contain high levels of vitamin C. Fresh-squeezed lemon or lime juice is a great way to start your morning. **Beets** are high in plant-flavonoids and beta-carotene, which increase liver health. **Apples** contain pectin and other chemicals that cleanse toxins from the digestive tract, lowering the burden on your liver. Oils such as **Olive Oil**, used in moderation provide a lipid base for absorbing toxins and helping dispose of them, further lowering the burden.

Vegetables: **Carrots** are also high in plant-flavonoids and beta-carotene, providing a similar boost as beets to liver functioning. **Leafy Green Vegetables** can be consumed in almost any form (raw, steamed, juiced), and neutralize many of the environmental toxins that tax our detoxification systems. They suck up heavy metals, chemicals and pesticides. They are an essential protective measure for the liver. **Bitter gourd, arugula, dandelion greens, spinach, mustard greens, and chicory** increase the creation and flow of bile, which facilitates the removal of waste. **Cruciferous Vegetables** such as **broccoli and cauliflower** increase circulating glucosinolate boosting the production of detox enzymes in the liver and lower the risk of cancer. **Cabbage** works in the same way.

Nuts, berries, and grains: **Avocados** are a super-food involved in the production of glutathione, a substance crucial to liver health. Eating avocados regularly is a great way to improve overall health. Some **Whole Grains** such as **Brown Rice** contain B-complex vitamins; they improve fat metabolization, liver function, and liver decongestion. If you're eating foods made with flour, be sure to choose whole grains rather than white flour. **Walnuts** help the liver detoxify ammonia and function normally through the amino acid arginine, glutathione, and omega-3 fatty acids. Chew the nuts completely (so that they are liquid in your mouth) before swallowing.

Artichoke, asparagus, kale, and Brussels sprouts are also great foods for liver health.

Recovery from degenerative diseases like Lyme requires liver cleanses as well as a liver-healthy diet. Simply eating the foods listed above is not enough to keep your liver healthy: you must perform a liver cleanse at least twice per year. If you do not, environmental toxins can stay trapped in your liver and stop you from being healthy again. According to many doctors, including Dr. Hulda Clark, Andreas Moritz, and Dr. Donald Monus (just to name a few), liver cleanses can improve digestion, and make allergies disappear. Many of your aches and pains will also be reduced, increasing energy and overall wellness. It is crucial, however, to perform a parasite and kidney cleanse before attempting the liver flush.

Flushing out the liver bile ducts is an incredible way to improve overall health. *"The liver has direct control over the growth and functioning of every cell in the body. Any kind of malfunctioning, deficiency, or abnormal growth pattern of the cell is largely due to poor liver performance. As misleading as this may be to the patient and his doctor, the origin of most diseases can easily be traced to the liver."*

Procedure:

Dr. Clark's Liver Flush

[Adapted from *The Cure for all Advanced Cancers*, by Hulda Clark, 1999 edition]

Before you Begin:

Dr. Clark suggests that you follow the rest of her program if you plan to perform this liver cleanse, especially the parasite killing program and the kidney cleanse. She further suggests that you ozonate the olive oil to prevent the proliferation of parasites or viruses that become dislodged during the cleanse. Be aware that the stones that you see may not be as large as you expected, and you may not see any parasites. Beginning the detoxification process can still aid in overall health and recovery.

What you'll need:

4 tbsp. Epsom salts

1/2 cup olive oil (ozonated for 20 minutes if possible)

2/3 cup of freshly squeezed grapefruit juice (from fresh pink grapefruit: "Hot wash twice first and dry each time.")

1 large plastic straw

A pint jar with a lid

10-20 drops of Black Walnut tincture (to kill parasites)

What to do:

You'll need to rest the day after the cleanse, so be sure to pick a day before you have a day off. Do not take any medicines that you can live without (including the ones from this program). Eat a very light breakfast like fruit or juice (avoid dairy). Do not eat anything after that to avoid feeling ill later.

At 2 PM: Mix 4 tbsp. of Epsom Salt with 3 cup water and pour the mixture into to your jar. Place the jar in the fridge (you may enjoy the taste more if it is cold).

At 6 PM: Drink ¾ cup of the mixture. If you can't tolerate the taste, you can add a little bit of vitamin C powder (1/8 tsp.) or simply drink a little bit of water or wash out your mouth.

At 8 PM: Drink another ¾ cup of the salt mixture and prepare for bed.

At 9:45 PM: Pour ½ cup of the olive oil into the jar. Use hot water to twice wash the grapefruit, then dry it and squeeze juice into a measuring cup. Use a fork to get rid of any remaining pulp. You should have between ½ and ¾ cup of grapefruit juice when you're finished (more is better). Add the juice to the jar, along with the Black Walnut tincture, close and shake the mixture until it becomes watery. Go to the bathroom a few times, but don't be more than 15 minutes late for the 10 PM part of the procedure.

10 PM: Drink the "potion". Use the straw to help yourself drink it. Drink it standing up, and finish it within five minutes ("very elderly or weak persons" are permitted an extension of 15 minutes). Lie down on your left side as soon as you finish the potion. Keep your head high on your pillow and lay perfectly still for 20 or more minutes. Picture the processes taking place in your liver. There should be no pain, but you might feel the stones moving through your bile ducts. Fall asleep (do not clean your kitchen or do any other chores).

After Waking (after 6 AM): Take the third dose of the Epsom salt mixture as long as you don't have any indigestion or nausea. You can go back to sleep afterwards.

2 Hours Later: Take the final dose of Epsom salts. If you want to, you can go back to sleep.

2 Hours Later: You can start drinking fruit juice now, and move on to solid fruit half an hour later. You can eat a light, regular meal within an hour. You should feel fine by evening.

Other Notes:

- You will most likely have diarrhea in the morning.

- Examine your excrement to find the gallstones. Count the approximate number of tan or green gallstones, because you need to pass 2000 stones to improve your health. The green suggests that they are from the liver. The tan stones may be "chaff" and getting rid of it is as important in the cleanse as getting rid of stones.

- You must repeat the cleanse to achieve results about every three weeks. Do not perform the cleanse if you are experiencing an acute illness.

- While you may feel ill for one or two days, that does not indicate that the cleanse is unsafe.

- Dr. Clark modified this recipe from an older one "invented hundreds, if not thousands, of years ago."

"This procedure contradicts many modern medical viewpoints. Gallstones are thought to be formed in the gallbladder, not the liver. They are thought to be few, not thousands. They are not linked to pains other than gallbladder attacks. It is easy to understand why this is thought: by the time you have acute pain attacks, some stones are in the gallbladder, are big enough and sufficiently calcified to see on X-ray, and have caused inflammation there. When the gallbladder is removed the acute attacks are gone, but the bursitis and other pains and digestive problems remain.

The truth is self-evident. People who have had their gallbladder surgically removed still get plenty of green, bile-coated stones, and anyone who cares to dissect their stones can see that the concentric circles and crystals of cholesterol match textbook pictures of "gallstones" exactly."

There are different methods of a liver/gallbladder flush by Hulda Clark, Andreas Moritz, Dr. Monus and others. I personally follow the instructions by Dr. Monus; they ALL WORK! I have done seven consequent flushes in a period of 6 months so far. I feel great after each flush. My energy skyrockets, my head becomes clear, a sense of well-being and joy takes place of mood swings. I am dedicated to using the flush technique until I have no more stones.

I did become sick three times out of the seven flushes until I learned my mistakes and found ways to trap the released toxins and prevent them from entering the blood stream.

Rule # 1:

Do NOT eat anything 16 hours before the flush! If you do—you will get sick and you will be vomiting after ingesting the oil/grapefruit juice mixture.

Rule # 2:

Take activated charcoal or any other detox supplement, containing activated charcoal and bentonite clay 30-40 minutes after oil/grapefruit juice mixture ingestion to trap the released toxins and prevent them from entering the blood stream.

Rule # 3:

Have your coffee enema handy! If you do get sick (fever, headache, sweats, racing heart rate – signs of high toxicity levels), have an enema right away! You might need to have 2 or more enemas to release all the toxins from your colon. You will feel relief right away and signs of sickness will be gone at a finger snap! Try to get a colonic after to make sure all toxins are flushed out!

"To permanently cure bursitis, back pain, allergies, or other health problems, and to prevent diseases from arising, you need to remove all the stones. This may require at least 8 to 12 flushes, which can be performed at three-week or monthly intervals. (Do not flush more frequently than that!)

The important thing to remember is that once you have started cleansing the liver, you should keep cleansing it until no more stones come out during two consecutive flushes. Leaving the liver half clean for a long period of time (three or more months) may cause greater discomfort than not cleansing it at all. The liver, as a whole, will begin to function more efficiently soon after the first flush, and you may notice sudden improvements, sometimes within several hours. Pains will lessen, energy will increase, and clarity of mind will improve considerably. However, within a few days, stones from the rear of the liver will have traveled 'forward' toward the two main bile ducts (hepatic ducts) in the liver, which may cause some or all of the previous symptoms of discomfort to return. In fact, you might feel disappointed because the recovery seems so short-lived. Yet all of this merely indicates that some stones were left behind and are ready to be removed with the next round of cleansing.

Nevertheless, the liver's self-repair and cleansing responses will have increased significantly, adding a great deal of effectiveness to this extremely important organ of the body. As long as there are still a few small stones traveling from some of the thousands of small bile ducts to any of the hundreds of larger bile ducts, they may combine to form larger stones and produce previously experienced symptoms, such as backache, headache, ear ache, digestive trouble, bloating, irritability, anger, and so forth, although these may be less severe than they were before.

If two consecutive new cleanses no longer produce any stones, which may happen after 6 to 8 flushes (in severe cases it may take 10 to 12 or more), your liver can be considered 'stone-free'. Nevertheless, it is recommended that you repeat the liver flush every six to eight months. Each flush will give a further boost to the liver and take care of any toxins or new stones that may have accumulated in the meantime.

Caution: *Never cleanse when you are suffering from an acute illness, even if it is just a simple cold. If you suffer from a chronic illness, however, cleansing your liver may be the best thing you can do for yourself."*

A liver flush is an absolute must; something you are supposed to repeat at least 3-6 times (if you are perfectly healthy)... and at least 6-10 times if you have any health problems, and more then 10-20 times if you are suffering from Allergies, CFS, MS, MCS, FMS, Eczema, Psoriasis, Acne, Cancer, Arthritis, Body Odor, Ulcerative Colitis... or any other chronic illness.

Real Cases:

I am writing to share a few words of encouragement with others out there. Before starting the parasite/candida cleanse and liver flush, I was experiencing problems of unexplained muscle pain, and terrible indigestion right after meals (usually containing fat). I was also experiencing what looked like a rash on my arms after eating. My doctor didn't know what to make of the symptoms. He diagnosed me with fibromyalgia and gave me pain medication and something to help me sleep at night. He told me that if I continued to experience problems after eating, that he would check to see if I was having gallbladder trouble. It was then that I found this wonderful web site! I have completed my 5th successful flush. The muscle pain is gone (no more pain medication is needed). What appears to have been food allergy reactions - is now down to a very mild reaction. The painful swelling around my ankles has also decreased. I may not be totally healed yet.............but am definitely well on the way to recovery. THIS WORKS!!!!!!

After 15 liver cleanses, 2025 stones have appeared.

All allergies are gone and I can eat anything I want to with one exception: MSG-which really isn't food anyways.

Rod

୬ ୭

I will do my 8th flush this weekend and I am absolutely amazed at how healthy I feel... I think my arthritis is gone too... I had a ruptured disc which was surgically removed in 1980... ever since then I have had a constant companion of chronic pain... but today even with all the rainy wet weather we've been having here... I have had absolutely no pain at all... absolutely unbelievable... it is so unreal... for the first time since surgery I am totally pain free... usually every time it rains I hurt the most... this is soooo coool...

Psoriasis is gone...

Cholesterol gone...

Thyroid problem... gone...

Hemorrhoid... gone...

and I think my arthritis is gone too...

Can't remember when I've felt so terrific... but I've been doing other things to help also... like diet... I've cut out meats... dairy products... refined food substances... and that seems to have helped a lot also... doing cayenne to improve circulation... I think perhaps it's the combination of things that is working... but certainly intend to keep doing what I've been doing and I can't help but believe I continue to keep getting better... only it seems hard to believe I could ever feel any better than I do right now...

It's a wonderful day in the neighborhood boys and girls...

;-)

Juice Fast

66Fasting is the greatest remedy
– the physician within. 99

Philippus Paracelsus

Ok my friends; I know what you are thinking! *"You have convinced me to do coffee enemas, get my guts cleaned out by a colon therapist, converted me into a raw vegan, made me do liver flushes and see tons of green colored stones in my poop, and now you want me to fast!? Are you out of your mind, girl?"*

Well, first of all let's call it a "juice flush" or even a "juice feast" instead of a fast. On a juice flush/feast you can drink as much juice as you can. Yes, you heard me right—as much as you can! You will literally flood your body with all the nutrients from raw, fresh squeezed juice and flush out all the toxins from your liver, kidneys, lungs, skin and the whole body!

Not only does juice fasting clean out your body, it also gives it more vitamins, minerals, phytochemicals, antioxidants, and enzymes. Juices from living fruits and vegetables have many healing properties. They also require almost no energy to digest, meaning that they heal without forcing your body to focus on them. They are low calorie, encouraging your body to pull apart nutrients and waste already in the body to maintain its energy. Juice fasting can improve vitality for almost everyone by altering cancer cells, toxins, built-up chemicals, excess fat, transformed fatty acids, and impacted mucus in the bowel.

When health begins to decline, usually the first thing people try are supplements or even worse pharmaceutical drugs. When one drug/supplement doesn't work, then a person usually tries another. And on and on it goes; the drug/supplement roller coaster. Each supplement is supposedly more "miraculous" than the other. Meanwhile, the truly powerful healing techniques such as juice fasting are ignored. Juice fasting is THE quickest, most effective way to heal from almost any health issue.

JUICING HELPS INCURABLE DISEASES:

Many doctors have used it as a healing technique for centuries for those with cancer, depression, arthritis, severe infections that failed with antibiotics, autoimmune diseases and many other supposedly incurable diseases. The results were nothing short of miraculous. I have personally met a woman that healed herself from 23 years of suffering from Lyme disease with a 21-day juice fast. She did not claim it was easy. She described her experience as her body "burned" all toxins, parasites, bacteria and viruses and it was making her extremely sick. She would have quit if it were not for her loving husband who took care of her and prepared juices for her and encouraged her to stay on a fast just a little longer when she was about to give up. This lady has been symptom-free for the past three years. Moreover, she had passed Lyme to her son in utero. When he was born, he was diagnosed autistic. For many years she felt guilty and blamed herself for her son's illness. After her recovery this woman realized how powerful diet and juice fasting was. She put her son on a raw vegan diet with lots of detox supplements. And guess what, her son recovered despite all medical prognoses!

This is how strong and effective a juicing program can be. And as effective as it is, I have found that combining it with a colon cleanse, moderate physical exercise, rebounding, yoga and stretches, daily sun exposure (without any sunscreen!), prayers, meditation, and visualization are all able to heal and reverse just about any incurable diseases.

"Juice fasting can produce immediate and dramatic improvement. I have seen results producing a 'cancer free' condition in as little as three weeks. I have no hard numbers to quote, but my observation and opinion is that those who diligently apply these principles have at least an 80% chance of complete remission in two months. Often a juice fasting procedure is all that is needed for successfully treating cancer. I have seen many people make complete recoveries from cancer by juicing alone." (Bob Davis who healed his prostate cancer by engaging in colon cleansing, detox diet & juice fasting.)

As cancer victim George Malkmus affirms, *"Many digestive systems are not functioning well and the sicker the person, the more difficult it is to digest and assimilate the nutrients in raw vegetables, because they contain the pulp or fiber. But with the pulp or fiber removed, the nutrients can pass directly into the blood stream and within minutes are feeding the cells and restoring the immune system."* George Malkmus healed himself of colon cancer by switching to a vegetarian regime composed largely of raw fruits and vegetables, amending his lifestyle and *"drinking lots of freshly extracted carrot juice."*

"...not only was my cancer gone, but so were all my other physical problems. These included high blood pressure, severe sinus and allergy problems, hemorrhoids, hypoglycemia, fatigue, pimples... even body odor and dandruff!"

George Malkmus writes that *"...Our body is a living organism made up of living cells, and living cells require living food (raw food) to function properly... the fastest way to restore the body to wellness is not through the eating of raw food alone, but also by consuming large quantities of raw, freshly-extracted vegetable juices. The juices do not heal. But what they do is provide the body with concentrated building materials so the body can heal itself. The first part of the body that will restore when given the proper nutrients is the immune system. As the immune system restores, then it seeks out the trouble spots throughout the body and starts to heal them. And it doesn't matter what the symptoms are, the body is self-healing when we stop the offense and provide the body cells with the proper building materials."*

Fasting is a great way to take control of your health, the natural way. It is an alternative choice that we all can make to heal our whole bodies without spending a dime on pharmaceutical drugs or risking the typical side effects of medication.

I understand that sometimes it is hard to stop eating and start your juice fast at home when no one supports you. I actually was not able to do it on my own. All my cleanses, I have done at health retreats where I was among like-minded people and had the support of amazing practitioners. It was always my dream to open up a clinic or a health retreat to help people prevent and reverse degenerative illnesses. My dream came true—after my full recovery I started a *Health Mastery Retreat*, where we take participants on a 7-day juice fast accompanied with colon therapy, coffee enemas, acupuncture, chiropractic adjustments, hyperthermia, and other natural treatments. I really encourage you to find a health retreat that will assist in your recovery.

Hyperthermia

Happy Juicing My Friends!

66Give me a chance to create a fever and I will cure any disease. 99

Ancient physician Parmenides

Yes, this is my favorite therapy! Hyperthermia simply means elevating your body's temperature. My favorites are Korean or Russian sauna and hot yoga. During my sick days I was sweating 5 times per week to detox, kill bacteria and viruses, and boost my immune system.

Your body uses fevers to return you to health. High temperatures speed up metabolism and stop viruses and bacteria from growing. It can help fight colds and other regular infections as well as complex health problems like polio and cancer. Hyperthermia is used to treat infectious diseases, rheumatic diseases, skin disorders, insomnia, muscle aches and pains, and even cancer. Modern medicine often thinks of fever as an uncomfortable symptom of illness, and reduces it using drugs like aspirin. In past eras, healers embraced fever as a method of extreme detox. If fever is an effective method of getting rid of disease, then we are preventing it from doing its job by taking these drugs. Sweat allows the body to get rid of toxins that the liver and kidneys would otherwise be forced to process. Even in healthy people, sweating can be a great way to shed toxins.

Hyperthermia may be commonly known as heat therapy, fever therapy, or sweat therapy. The heat works by cleaning out clogged pores, killing bacteria and viruses, increasing circulation and otherwise enhancing the immune system. It increases metabolism, circulation, tissue rebuilding/healing and valuable cellular activity. Much like a heating pad, it can help heal injuries. It stimulates vital body functions. Fever is very effective and all natural. Inducing a fever taps into the natural healing process for killing viruses and bacteria.

Many physiological actions take place in the body in response to the raised temperature. The viruses, bacteria, and parasites wreaking havoc on your body cannot tolerate the same range of temperatures as your body can, so raising the temperature kills them but not your body. This applies to Borrelia, Bartonella, rhinovirus, HIV, the microorganisms responsible for syphilis and gonorrhea, just to name a few. In situations where not all of the invading organisms are killed, their numbers are still reduced and the immune system is stimulated. When you have a fever, your body produces antibodies and interferon which kills the viruses and stops them from reproducing. Hyperthermia can also help detox your system by tapping into the toxins stored in fat.

Hot baths have also been used to treat herpes simplex and shingles, as well as the flu, the common cold, Chronic Fatigue Syndrome, and other illnesses. Use of hot baths is supported by N.D.'s at the Bastyr College Natural Health Clinic. The treatment may initially exacerbate symptoms, but after a short time improves patients' lives. Other Seattle practitioners, such as Bruce Milliman, induce fevers to treat CFS. Patients have three fevers a day for three weeks, during which they stay home and get total bed rest. Fevers are induced by soaking patients in a bath of water as hot as they can tolerate while consuming 2000 mg of vitamin C combined with 12 oz. of water. The person undergoing treatment leaves the bath after five minutes, then gets into a specially prepared hot bed, staying under flannel and wool blankets for 20 minutes with a hot water bottle under the breast (on women) or above the liver (on men). This method pushes the body to sweat as it tries to return to normal temperature, promoting detoxification and the other benefits of a fever. Milliman has had a 70-75% success rate with "turning up the thermostat" when patients remain in the procedure for the entire time.

Dr. Lewis has also had good results treating Chronic Fatigue Syndrome with hyperthermia. For certain cases, Dr. Lewis prescribes hyperthermia as a form of self-care. In one instance, he suggested a patient take hot tub treatments at home three to four times weekly. *"During the following year,"* Dr. Lewis reports, *"...her condition improved wonderfully. While not fully recovered, her energy level is substantially higher, and she credits this to her hot tub routine."*

Studies have found that hyperthermia treatments play a role in stimulating the immune system. After treatment, the number of white blood cells drops and then increases dramatically in number and efficiency. Substances like interleukin (implicated in immune functioning) increase after treatment. Dr. A.C. Guyton, M.D. states that metabolic rate increases as temperature increases, which may be related to an increase in immune functioning.

Many viral infections have been successfully treated at the Natural Health Clinic of Bastyr College using hyperthermia. It can help in cases where natural and traditional treatments have not been very helpful. After starting hyperthermia treatments, patients may see immediate results, though their ability to tolerate higher temperatures improves as time goes on. As a part of the *Healing Aids Research Project*, the Clinic included hyperthermia treatment in its investigation of treatments for HIV because it can stimulate the immune system, and aid in detoxification. Some research found that HIV becomes inactive when exposed to higher and higher temperatures.

On my way to recovery I was sweating 5 times per week – either hot yoga or Russian and Korean sauna. I know for 100% it was one of the MAJOR therapies on my way to recovery. To this day I continue practicing hot yoga several times a week and I visit the sauna several times per month.

For those of you who cannot tolerate heat, start slowly or use infrared sauna. Traditional saunas are a high heat, low humidity environment. Temperatures range between 80-90°C (185-195°F) and water is splashed over the heater rocks to create a blast of hyper-steam and intensify the feeling of heat. For those who enjoy this experience, there is nothing in the world quite like it.

Infrared saunas may provide an alternative for those who want to try saunas but can't or those who simply don't enjoy them. These saunas are enjoyable in their own right, but aren't the same as traditional saunas. They are milder than conventional saunas, as they work by heating the body first and the air second.

REAL CASE:

I have never felt so alive and I am young and never thought I was unhealthy. I haven't had any cold symptoms, headaches or any minor problems since using sauna and ridding the toxins.

I am using the sauna 5/7 days/week. I just love it. There are now some mornings when I wake up and feel no pain in my

Hydrotherapy

CONTRAST SHOWERS

neck and shoulders. I look forward to more days like this.

"The more severe the pain or illness, the more severe will be the necessary changes. These may involve breaking bad habits, or acquiring some new and better ones. **"**

Peter McWilliams

Finnish, Latvian, and Russian people have old traditions of taking a sauna then performing some kind of cold immersion or plunge pool. Contrast showers use the same methods for people who may not have access to saunas and plunge pools, and encourage gradual adjustment between more extreme temperatures.

Contrast shower is a MUST for me every single morning! No excuses! Even when I am travelling and I am not able to perform all of my morning rituals, a shower is available everywhere! Contrast shower is one of my favorite rituals and therapies, besides increasing circulation and boosting the immune system, a contrast shower leaves me feeling energized and alive!

Using different temperatures of water provides many

of the same benefits as hyperthermia: it increases circulation through various tissues, allowing better nutrition and waste disposal to take place, encourages deep detoxification, and increases overall immune functioning. It can even increase white blood cell count. The hot and cold water serve different functions, and together form a strong defense for your body.

When applied in short-bursts, the cold water decreases inflammation, helps keep you alert, and reduces constipation. Longer applications can raise strength and resistance to disease as well. Short applications of hot water cause small blood vessels to dilate, relaxes muscles overall and raises body temperature. In long form, applications can help eliminate toxins and encourage healing. As many of us know, water can help us relax and stay calm, as well as reduce pain. Avoid applications of hot water when treating an acute inflammatory problem.

You can try hydrotherapy in your next shower! Use hot water for three minutes, then 30 seconds of cold water, and repeat three times each shower. Be sure to end on cold water to leave you feeling invigorated and fresh.

I just love the way my favorite Dr. Schulze describes hydrotherapy. Many, many years ago he wanted to investigate hydrotherapy, so he went down to one of the last operating hydrotherapy clinics in the United States. (Dr. Schulze clarifies, that he went to a hard-core hydrotherapy *clinic, not a posh-lush spa*!) He wanted to experience the healing power of these great old treatments that existed years ago, before they disappeared. By the way, this miraculous healing therapy went out of *vogue in* America in the last century because it involved nudity, not because it did not work! In fact, it is still extremely popular in many other countries where the people live much longer and much healthier than they do in the United States.

When Dr. Schulze walked up to the clinic, he was more than astonished. There were elderly people sitting all over the porch with their heads down , looking stunned, dazed and doped-up, almost drooling on the floor. It looked like a sanitarium for the brain dead, but he still wanted to see what, if anything, they offered.

So he went in and asked for the *full hydrotherapy* treatment. And he got what he asked for! They put him in a hot tub and made him drink hot water. Then they took him out and put him in a shower where cold water jets hit him all over the body. Then he went to another hot tub and steam bath. Then they put him in a room and applied hot packs and ice packs all over his body. After that they laid him down on another bed for a few minutes. Finally, they put him in a wheel chair and wheeled him out to the front, where he sat with all these other people staring at the floor with drool coming out of his mouth. Now he realized that these people were not brain dead; there was nothing wrong with them. They were *relaxed, physically blissed out - emotionally and spiritually healed.*

You can find hydrotherapy clinics all over Europe, Russia, and Asia. As you already know, any treatment that "big pharma" cannot profit from, is not approved in the US. Now the good news... you do not have to travel overseas for this miraculous healing modality, you can perform this therapy in the comfort of your own shower!

A last inspirational story on contrast showers; it does become more tolerable and even pleasurable over time. When I started I was able to do one round only. Then slowly I began adding rounds. Now I am able to tolerate cold water for a long time and it does not really shock my body anymore. I actually love the energy and vibrancy I am getting from the cold water and every morning I am looking forward to it!

<u>REAL CASE:</u>

Recently I have just started taking cold showers. Now after 3 months, my mood and health feel incredible! I'm addicted to cold showers, they feel so refreshing and relaxing, it feels like I'm under a waterfall. Before I started taking cold showers, I used to suffer from fatigue and after the first cold shower my mood and health feel 100%.

Bec B from Victoria

Dry Skin Brushing

" *He's the best physician that knows the worthlessness of the most medicines.* **"**

Benjamin Franklin

Dry skin brushing --- I just **LOVE** this procedure! It makes me feel so good like a mini massage. And I promise – you will love it too! This ritual comes between rebounding and a contrast shower in the morning. I was introduced to dry skin brushing in my immunology class during acupuncture school. It is a technique that I have used throughout the years and I can attest, that when I do it regularly, I notice health improvements as well as glowing skin.

Your skin is more than just a protective barrier; it's also one of the most important organs that helps detoxify your body. It gets rid of nearly two pounds of toxins every day. What you put on your skin matters: many beauty products, deodorants, clothes, or even soaps can stop your skin from being healthy, and pull toxicity into your system. Keeping your skin healthy can help reduce the burden on other detoxification systems, like your lungs, liver, and kidneys. Skin problems are not superficial, and may be an indicator of your body's overall ability to detoxify.

Dry skin brushing supports your skin as it detoxifies. Many people find it energizing, and it can help prevent and reduce illness by providing immune support. Dry brushing every morning unblocks pores and prevents dead skin from building up. It also aids your body in disposing of metabolic waste, allowing it to focus on fighting bacteria. The procedure can feel luxurious, and helps the lymphatic system function at its best. Lymph is one of your body's support systems, located between the cells in all tissues. Like blood, it provides nourishment and collects waste. Brushing your skin prevents blockages of this system.

While your circulatory system is motivated by your heart, lymph can become clogged without regular exercise. As you experience more and more infections, lymphatic systems become bogged down with dead cell bodies. People who have chronic diseases are especially prone to coagulated lymph. By brushing, stretching, and exercising, we can breakdown and prevent blockages, encouraging your body to make more white blood cells and better fight of infections. It can also help you look healthier by improving the condition of your skin, and allows oil glands to naturally protect and moisturize your skin.

Advice:
- Use a brush with natural bristles and a long handle.
- Do not over brush. Brushing once a day will work for most people. Don't brush over open or inflamed places in your skin, as this will only exacerbate the problem.

- Try brushing first thing in the morning before a shower 5-6 days a week. Mornings are a good time for brushing and stretching because it increases alertness and helps prevent toxins that build up during sleep from becoming a problem.

- Always brush towards your heart because lymph flows upward. Follow this pattern: Feet, legs, back, stomach, chest, arms, underarms, back of the neck, top of the chest, then lightly on the sides of the neck. Avoid the nipples.

Oil Pulling Therapy

66A wise man should consider that health is the greatest of human blessings, and learn how by his own thought to derive benefit from his illnesses. 99

Hippocrates

FROM MY INBOX:

I was fortunate to find out about Dr Karach's oil pulling therapy over 16 years ago, and my objective was to improve my immune system, as a preventative. And it certainly has done so, for example, the number of colds has gone down a lot. Plus, my digestion has improved very much. Also, I can go on for more hours without feeling the need to eat.

Basically, my opinion is that oil pulling is one of the very best ways to stimulate the body's natural healing abilities, and that includes detoxification. 15-20 minutes in the morning of oil pulling regularly, while taking a shower or shaving or ... - is one of the wisest things we could do, health wise.

❧   ❧

I came down with fibromyalgia last year and I know all about the pain you are experiencing. I decided I would continue do-

ing my Ayurvedic practice of "oil pulling" - and it reversed the disease. I don't know what it can do for you but there are many insiders in the pharmaceutical industry that have broken ranks about the effectiveness of pain killer treatments and hematological interventions. They simply don't work. This remedy however reversed many illnesses for me which the medical profession could not treat; many people have found relief from this practice. I don't know how chronic or pernicious your disease is, mine got cured within a matter of days. I have found this remedy to be wonderful. The reason why it is not adequately promoted is because it does not cost anything and can't be patented. I hope you find some relief soon. This method took away my pain in a matter of days. Don't know whether it may work but you can always give it a try.

Chronic diseases that you have had for a while take longer to cure. I had lived with CFS also for over a decade, complete exhaustion, no energy at all. The oil pulling reversed it in under a week. You might also like to go to www.curezone.com and check the oil pulling forum. I can't guarantee anything, but neither can those doctors! I have an e-friend interstate who is in excruciating pain with Fibro. She went down the conventional route and lives with brain fog, sleepless nights and agony. She can barely type on a computer and her husband has to drive her to work.

Just go to the health food store and get sunflower oil and also some sesame oil for your supply. They must be cold pressed. Just pick one bottle and start your practice when you are through with one bottle after a month or so, rotate and go onto the next one. Sunflower and sesame are the two that are the most effective.

This practice is old, it is found in the Vedas, and you will be encouraged by the results. I hope you are successful with this therapy, as I know the pain you are experiencing. I know a lot about the industry and what they do too. Just approach your oil pulling as you would any other treatment, see what happens. I hope you are cured I really do, this was the only thing that worked for me. You may also like to look at www. earthclinic.com and check out the posts on oil pulling.

❧ ❧

Chronic illnesses are difficult to treat, I don't know whether it will work for you but it has reversed so many things for me and I am being honest with you I am not a doctor but am an ardent proponent of this method because of what it did. It saved my life when doctors couldn't help me. Just make sure you follow the directions correctly and do it right.

You may like to be on the computer checking e-mails while you are swishing, that is a good way to pass the time. If it cures you it will make me a very happy lady as I have lived with illness all my life, so I know your predicament. Good luck I really hope that it may offer you something. It can't hurt to try, give it a week or so, maybe swishing several times a day to intensify the effect. They have a forum on www.curezone.com for oil pulling so you can be in regular dialog with a community and people will gladly answer your questions. Follow the protocol, it is easy to do. I wish you well and sincerely hope you can put this behind you, it could possibly take longer than a month, and there are no guarantees, just try it and see. I hope you are cured and go back to living a normal life.

❧ ❧

I had heard about oil-pulling therapy (OP) from my healer, same lady that introduced me to "Two Feathers", Multi-Wave-Oscillator, Ondamed, and other healing wonders. I was very skeptical at first and did not really take it seriously. Only a year later, during my extensive research of holistic healing, I learned about OP and became very confident in the potency of this treatment. I bought and read a book called, *Oil Pulling Therapy: Detoxifying and Healing the*

Body through Oral Cleansing by Bruce Fife and all I wished was that I had been more open-minded to try OP a year earlier.

According to an article on the Earth Clinic website, Oil Pulling is reported to cure: *"Mouth & Gum Disease; Stiff Joints; Allergies; Asthma; High Blood Sugar; Constipation; Migraines; Bronchitis; Eczema; Heart, Kidney, Lung Diseases; Leukemia; Arthritis; Meningitis; Insomnia; Menopause (hormonal issues); Cancer; AIDS; Chronic Infections; Varicose Veins; High Blood Pressure; Diabetes; Polio; Cracked Heels."*

Or as Dr. Karach, one of the biggest proponents of oil pulling says, *"The Oil-therapy heals totally headaches, bronchitis, tooth pain, thrombosis, eczema, ulcers, intestinal diseases, heart and kidney diseases, encephalitis and woman's diseases. Preventively the growth of malignant tumors is cut and healed. Chronic blood diseases, paralysis, diseases of nerves, stomach, lungs and liver and sleeplessness are cured."*

First explained in antiquity, this Ayurvedic technique was promoted by Deepak Chopra in *Perfect Health*. Regular use will help you purify and strengthen your body. Before you eat or brush your teeth in the morning, use a small amount (up to1 tbsp.) of cold pressed oil the way you would mouthwash, but for 10 to 20 minutes. Finding the oil that works best for you comes down to your own tastes, and some possibilities are sesame, sunflower, coconut, flaxseed, walnut, olive, and grapeseed oil.

Oil pulling is a very simple process:

Take one tablespoon of oil (sesame or coconut) in the mouth in the morning before breakfast on an empty stomach. Move oil back and forth in the mouth as rinsing or swishing for fifteen to twenty minutes. Dr Karach explains it as, *"sip, suck and pull through the teeth."* When you swish oil thoroughly it mixes with saliva and activates the enzymes. Enzymes are one of the most interesting and important substances found in nature. They draw toxins out of the blood. Make sure never to swallow the oil because it becomes toxic. During the oil swishing the oil gets thinner and white, even kind of foamy. If the oil is still yellow, it has not been pulled long enough. After about 20 minutes, spit the oil out. Make sure to wash your mouth thoroughly with filtered water.

The oil pulling therapy is done best before breakfast. To accelerate the healing process, it can be repeated three times a day, but always before meals on an empty stomach. When you first begin oil pulling (OP) allow yourself to do it in shorter intervals in the beginning so that you can acclimate. If performed correctly, the oil will become thin and white before you spit it out. You may want to spit into the toilet or a compost heap rather than the sink. Remember, once you have spit, you should rinse your mouth with water or salt water, or brush your teeth with baking soda. Drink a glass of water to fully clean your mouth.

This method works for multiple reasons. Some sources believe that it will draw toxins out of your teeth and mucus membranes. Ayurveda suggests that the tongue contains many connections to organs, as it is one of main key places in your body. Practitioners of Ayurveda use the tongue as a crucial part of their diagnostic repertoire. Still other viewpoints suggest that the oil itself has nutritional, antiviral, and anti-inflammatory properties, as oils with numerous benefits, such as sesame oil, are often used for this practice. The nutrients may be absorbed through the mouths mucous membranes.

A study conducted in a Dental College in India discovered that two weeks of this practice can significantly remove bad bacteria, leading to reduced levels of Streptococcus mutans, plaque and changes in gingival index. Many types of bacteria inhabit your mouth, and some form plaque which allows the development of many health problems. Buildup of plaque at the gum line can lead to large gaps between your gums and teeth which then become infected and cause major health crises. As pockets of your gums become infected, they can cause a chronic inflammatory response encouraging your body to cannibalize tissues and bone. Periodontitis emerges as the pockets deepen. We have already discussed the importance of dental health and the danger of root canals and cavitations earlier. This is more proof of the significance and relevance of OP. This connection suggests that OP can help with joint pain, arthritis, migraines, sinus infections, skin disorders, allergies, digestive issues, and many more issues. Periodontitis may increase risk of rheumatoid arthritis, respiratory disease, diabetes, Alzheimer's, and heart disease and encourage teeth to become loosened from the gums.

If you think about how often you swallow your saliva, it's pretty easy to figure out the many ways dental infection can spread through your body, especially when you include the other methods of spreading discussed with root canals and dental amalgams. Many of the bacteria you swallow produce exotoxins and endotoxins that cannot be processed by your stomach or immune system. These toxins are incredibly potent because they disrupt your cellular metabolism. Some can even kill you, such as botulinum, which is excreted by Clostridium botulinum. Exotoxins, such as lipopolysaccharide (LPS) can lead to endotoxic shock by confusing your immune system and encouraging inflammation. Many of these toxins are absorbed through the capillaries and mucous membranes in your mouth before even reaching your stomach or intestinal tract. This way, they go directly into your bloodstream constantly feeding you toxins. This constitutes a chronic infection, and causes illness. OP is crucial for preventing this catastrophe.

Happy oil pulling my friends!

Heliotherapy

66As I see it, every day you do one of two things:
build health or produce disease in yourself. **99**

Adelle Davis

This is not some fancy new expensive therapy; this is
one of nature's oldest secrets to health. Take advantage
of one of the cheapest, most available therapies around,
Heliotherapy! The sun brings renewed energy to the
earth and all of life. Learn just how good this free, natural resource is for you.

Sunlight is the source of all life on earth. We too thrive
in natural light and the sun's life-giving energy lifts our
physical and emotional vitality while improving our
well-being and health.

We're always hearing how we should avoid too
much sun. But, it is actually a vital element in both
physical and emotional health. A lack of adequate natural sun light compromises immunity and skeletal health
and can interfere with natural sleeping patterns. Various studies have shown the link between insufficient
natural light and depression during winter when natural light levels are low. In fact, insufficient sunlight

rather than too much is the greater contributor to ill health in our modern, indoor lifestyles.

Since the dawn of time up until the past two-hundred years, people lived and worked outdoors in the light of the sun. Now, we wake up in our homes, get in our car and drive to the office. For most of us, the only time we spend outdoors is simply walking back and forth to our vehicles. We make this even worse by wearing sunglasses which keep our eyes from receiving any of the sun's beneficial rays.

People have sunbathed to improve their lives since antiquity, where people often treated the sun with great reverence, as if it were a god. Depictions of sunbathing have been uncovered from ancient Greece, Egypt, Rome, Assyria, Babylon, and Persia. In Egypt, Babylon and Assyria, people maintained sun-gardens. By 200 AD, Mithraism, or sun worship, was nearly universal. The Romans believed that sunbaths would strengthen their gladiators, while physicians declared the sun "the best food and medicine in the world." Christianity, however, declared that sunbathing was sinful, and cracked down on sunbathing for a millennium.

Dr. G.D. Babbit, in agreement with the ancient Romans, notes that sunlight does indeed provide nutrition such as iron, magnesium, sodium, carbon and other important elements. He asks, *"But why shall we not take these elements in their ordinary form from our drugstores, and not go to the trouble of taking sun-baths? Because when these elements are given to us in so refined a form, as to come directly from the sun as an ether, or to float skywards and be driven to us by the solar rays, they must be far more penetrating, enduring, safe, pleasant, and upbuilding to the mental system than if they were used in a crude form."*

Dr. Babbit, isn't the only modern doctor to believe that

sunlight can prevent disease. Thorwald Madsen, a research scientist, has found that levels of disease increase as the amount of sun goes down. It has been used to treat tuberculosis (TB) since the late 1800's, when scientists discovered that TB and inflammation of the bones, joints and skin was greatly reduced by exposure to the sun. When children who had grown up in newly crowded and polluted urban centers spent time in the sun, their levels of vitamin D increased, helping them fight the disease. Prolonged exposure to sunlight can kill the TB causing bacteria, leading to amazing recoveries.

I would like to refer to one of my favorites books again, *Roger's Recovery from AIDS* by Bob Owen. A guy named Roger was deadly ill with AIDS and was given anywhere from 1 to 4 months to live. In just 30 days Roger had a complete turn around and regained his health back by not poisoning his body with processed foods and going on a juice fast. And guess what one of the major therapies on his way to recovery was? I hope you got it! It was heliotherapy! Roger was to sunbathe for 30 minutes on each side every single day in order to win his life back.

"The sun is needed for life. If you do not spend time in the sun you will be sick. The sun is vital for health, longevity, and to be disease free. If you are sick, one of the things you must do is get out in the sun. I can tell you this, that the sun itself can virtually cure disease." Kevin Trudeau

Let's just take a look at some of the major benefits of sunbathing:

BOOST IMMUNITY

The sun has a broad immune-boosting effect. It stimulates our pituitary gland - the master switch of our endocrine system. This produces hormones which determine the strength and speed of our body's immune responses.

Vitamin D, made by our body in response to sun exposure, helps white blood cells and the cells lining our respiratory tract fight off bacteria. And vitamin D also causes immune cells to migrate to the skin where they directly fight free-radical damage.

BEAT DEPRESSION AND INSOMNIA

Our pineal gland controls our sleep/wake cycles by secreting the hormone melatonin which stimulates our body to sleep. Many people need more sleep and are prone to depression especially during the winter because of increased melatonin production. Sunlight keeps us awake by inhibiting melatonin production and sun exposure during the day helps reset our body clock enabling a good night's sleep.

BOOST ENERGY

Better sleep and a sunny day naturally enhance energy levels. For the same reasons people tend to sleep more in winter – increased melatonin - lack of sunlight makes us drowsy throughout. A walk in the park at sunrise helps wake us up and get our day off to a good start. Even on a cloudy day, this natural light will give most of us the boost we need.

PROTECT YOUR SKIN

In addition to helping fight free-radical damage, sun exposure also stimulates the production of melanin - the brown pigment in our skin. Studies show that this pigment protects against skin cancer. Even people with fair skin can benefit if they build up pigmentation slowly over time.

STRENGTHEN BONES

Vitamin D is also needed for bone health. It stimulates and enhances absorption of calcium from our diet into our bones. Sunscreen blocks the synthesis of vitamin D and thus the benefits of natural light in addition to exposing our skin to toxic chemicals included in many commercial products.

The sun's warming rays aid recovery from stress and exertion. The warmth of healing sunlight deeply penetrates our skin, stimulating recuperative activities in our body including tissue repair, hormone synthesis and nutrient absorption. This also contributes to improved immunity and increased energy.

People who practice sunbathing have shown dramatically lowered blood pressure, regulated blood sugar, lowered cholesterol and an increased white blood cell count. Heliotherapy can make you much healthier, despite the cautions of modern scientists. The sun accelerates your body. Eating well can help minimize the ill effects of excessive sun exposure, while eating poorly will make your sunbathing less effective or even dangerous. If your diet is imperfect, use a little more caution when sunbathing to make sure you don't do any damage.

In principle, sunbathing is simple: you just lie out in the sun. Still, helpful tips and tricks will help you maximize befits and minimize harm.

- Use moderation when sunbathing, as moderation is always preferable to excess.

- During summer, sunbathing in the morning (9 AM- 11 AM) can be more effective than sunbathing in the mid-afternoon, because the type of light is better for you. Ultraviolet morning rays are very helpful, while mid-afternoon infrared can be damaging and too hot.

- During winter, the mornings are too cold, so sunbathe during midday for the most beneficial rays and temperature.

- Do not wear sunglasses, because they will prevent you from fully processing the light.

- Do not use sunscreen! The FDA does not allow natural forms of sunscreen (except those containing zinc oxide and titanium dioxide). Any conventional sunscreen will contain fragrance chemicals, parabens, alcohols, toxic solvents, and petroleum oils. Many of these ingredients have been linked to cancer, and constitute a "chemical assault" on your body. Sunscreen can limit the benefits of sunbathing by blocking the production of vitamin D, encouraging widespread vitamin deficiency and cancer, infections, depression, osteoporosis, and hormonal imbalances.

- Add antioxidants and super-foods to your diet to improve your resilience to the sun and reduce your burn time.

I'm a great example of this, actually, as I used to burn in just 30 - 40 minutes of sunlight when I was on an average western diet for years consuming lots of processed foods, processed sugars, and not enough nutrients. But now, as someone who eats mostly a raw vegan diet, supplementing with "superfoods" such as kale, broccoli, wheatgrass, barley grass and other greens, chia seeds, flax seeds and fresh veggie juices every day, I can spend hours in the sun and will not burn or peel after.

I personally have not worn sunscreen in over 5 years. I spend a large amount of time in the sun every day (running on the beach, playing tennis, hiking) since we get nearly 365 sunny days a year in San Diego, and I have absolutely no concerns whatsoever about skin cancer. Moreover, my skin, most friends tell me, looks significantly younger than my biological age. That's not from fancy skin care, facials, skin peels, creams, lotions and potions. As a matter of fact I do not put anything on my skin except coconut oil. My skin looks healthy and radiant from proper nutrition and hydration. Sun exposure does not make you "age" if you follow a clean, high-nutritional density and low processed-foods diet.

UV exposure alone does not cause skin cancer! It is a complete medical myth that *"UV exposure causes skin cancer."* This false idea is a total fabrication by the ignorant medical community (dermatologists) and the profit-driven sunscreen companies.

The truth is actually more complicated: Skin cancer can only be caused when UV exposure is combined with chronic nutritional deficiencies that create skin vulnerabilities.

To create skin cancer, in other words, you have to eat a junk food diet, avoid protective antioxidants, and then also experience excessive UV exposure. All three of those elements are required. Conventional medicine completely ignores the dietary influences and focuses entirely on just one factor: Sunscreen vs. no sunscreen. This is a one-dimensional approach to the issue that's grossly oversimplified to the point of being misleading.

"It is important to sunbathe and get sun over your entire body. Remember; never ever, ever use any sunscreen. Do not put anything on your skin that you can't eat. Sunscreens cause skin cancer." Kevin Trudeau

Not all "natural" sunscreen products are really natural.

While there are some good ones out there, many are just examples of *greenwashing*, where they use terms like "natural" or "organic" but still contain loads of synthetic chemicals anyway.

A good guide for checking on sunscreen products is the Environmental Working Group guide (EWG) at:

www.ewg.org/skindeep

Don't use any sunscreen product containing ingredients that sound like chemicals:

- Methyl...
- Propyl...
- Butyl...
- Ethyl...
- Trieth...
- Dieth...

etc.

A typical sunscreen product is made with over a dozen cancer-causing fragrance chemicals, and they're absorbed right through your skin. Most sunscreens, when applied as directed, are really just toxic chemical baths that heavily burden your liver and can give you cancer.

This is the truth about sunscreen that both the sunscreen industry and the cancer industry don't want you to hear. It's the dirty little secret of sunscreen: The more you use, the more you CAUSE cancer in your body! (And the more money the cancer centers make "treating" your cancer with yet even more deadly chemicals known as *chemotherapy*.)

So buyers beware. Sunscreen products are a minefield of lies, fraud and disinformation designed to keep you ignorant of the importance of sun exposure as well as the health risks associated with using cancer-causing chemicals on your skin.

Learn more about sunlight and vitamin D with these two resources:

FREE report: The truth about sunlight and vitamin D (*www.naturalnews.com/rr-sunlight.html*)

Learn more: (*www.naturalnews.com/032815_sunscreen_chemicals.html#ixzz1zLdaBJVX*)

There is one more very powerful healing benefit from the sun known as "sun gazing". The practice of sungazing practically resembles its name. At sunrise and sunset, when the sun is closest to the earth, sungazers stand barefoot on the earth and look directly at the sun for 10 seconds. The sun is the force of all life, and staring at it can saturate the whole body with large amounts of energy. They say sungazing benefits go even beyond sunbathing.

Please do your own research, use your common sense. Sungazing can be done right after sunrise or right before sunset ONLY. Do not stare at the sun other times; it can be dangerous for your eyes.

Stop Your Sugar Addiction NOW

❝Every form of addiction is bad, no matter whether the narcotic be alcohol or morphine or idealism. ❞

Carl Gustav Jung

If you make ONLY one change in your diet, let it be to eliminate processed sugar in any form and way.

Death by sugar may not be an overstatement — evidence is mounting that sugar is THE MAJOR FACTOR causing obesity and chronic disease. Sugar feeds cancer cells, triggers weight gain, and promotes premature aging.

Science has now shown us, beyond any shadow of a doubt, that sugar in your food, in all its myriad of forms, is taking a devastating toll on your health. The single largest source of calories for Americans comes from sugar — specifically high fructose corn syrup. Just take a look at the sugar consumption trends of the past 300 years:

- In 1700, the average person consumed about 4 pounds of sugar per year.

- In 1800, the average person consumed about 18 pounds of sugar per year.

- In 1900, individual consumption had risen to 90 pounds of sugar per year.

- In 2009, more than 50 percent of all Americans consume one-half pound of sugar PER DAY — translating to a whopping 180 pounds of sugar per year!

Sugar is loaded into your soft drinks, fruit juices, sports drinks, and hidden in almost all processed foods — from bologna to pretzels to Worcestershire sauce to cheese spread. And now most infant formula has the sugar equivalent of one can of Coca-Cola, so babies are being metabolically poisoned from day one if taking formula.

Sugar even in small amounts is detrimental. Just two teaspoons of sugar (far less than a typical soda or a bowl of cereal) has a significant hormonal and nutritional impact for several hours, throwing the body out of balance and into a state of biochemical chaos. If you eat sugar for breakfast, lunch, and dinner, your body remains in chaos all day, every day! You might say that you rarely or even never add any sugar to your food. Well, if you eat any baked goods – muffins, croissants, bagels, and breakfast cereals for breakfast – you eat SUGAR! If you add any ketchup, mustard, conventional salad dressings, balsamic vinegar, soups, dinner rolls, and the list goes on and on – you eat SUGAR!

Dr. William Coda Martin classified refined sugar as a poison because it has been depleted of its life forces, vitamins and minerals. *"What is left consists of pure, refined carbohydrates. The body cannot utilize this refined starch and carbohydrate unless the depleted proteins, vitamins and minerals are present. Nature supplies these elements in each plant in quantities sufficient to metabolize the carbohydrate in that particular plant. There is no excess for other added carbohydrates. Incomplete carbohydrate metabolism results in the formation of 'toxic metabolite' such as pyruvic acid and abnormal*

sugars containing five carbon atoms. Pyruvic acid accumulates in the brain and nervous system and the abnormal sugars
in the red blood cells. These toxic metabolites interfere with the
respiration of the cells. They cannot get sufficient oxygen to
survive and function normally. In time, some of the cells die.
This interferes with the function of a part of the body and is the
beginning of degenerative disease."

"Refined sugar is lethal when ingested by humans because
it provides only that which nutritionists describe as 'empty' or
'naked' calories. It lacks the natural minerals which are present
in the sugar beet or cane.

In addition, sugar is worse than nothing because it drains
and leaches the body of precious vitamins and minerals through
the demand its digestion, detoxification and elimination makes
upon one's entire system. So essential is balance to our bodies
that we have many ways to provide against the sudden shock of
a heavy intake of sugar. Minerals such as sodium (from salt),
potassium and magnesium (from vegetables), and calcium
(from the bones) are mobilized and used in chemical transmu-
tation; neutral acids are produced which attempt to return the
acid-alkaline balance factor of the blood to a more normal state.

Sugar taken every day produces a continuously over-acidic
condition, and more and more minerals are required from deep
in the body in the attempt to rectify the imbalance. Finally, in
order to protect the blood, so much calcium is taken from the
bones and teeth that decay and general weakening begin. Excess sugar eventually affects every organ in the body. Initially,
it is stored in the liver in the form of glucose (glycogen). Since
the liver's capacity is limited, a daily intake of refined sugar
(above the required amount of natural sugar) soon makes the
liver expand like a balloon. When the liver is filled to its maximum capacity, the excess glycogen is returned to the blood in
the form of fatty acids. These are taken to every part of the body
and stored in the most inactive areas: the belly, the buttocks,
the breasts and the thighs.

When these comparatively harmless places are completely filled, fatty acids are then distributed among active organs, such as the heart and kidneys. These begin to slow down; finally their tissues degenerate and turn to fat. The whole body is affected by their reduced ability, and abnormal blood pressure is created. The parasympathetic nervous system is affected; and organs governed by it, such as the small brain, become inactive or paralyzed. (Normal brain function is rarely thought of as being as biologic as digestion.) The circulatory and lymphatic systems are invaded, and the quality of the red corpuscles starts to change. An overabundance of white cells occurs, and the creation of tissue becomes slower. Our body's tolerance and immunizing power becomes more limited, so we cannot respond properly to extreme attacks; whether it is cold, heat, mosquitoes or microbes.

Excessive sugar has a strong mal-effect on the functioning of the brain. The key to orderly brain function is glutamic acid, a vital compound found in many vegetables. The B vitamins play a major role in dividing glutamic acid into antagonistic-complementary compounds which produce a 'proceed' or 'control' response in the brain. B vitamins are also manufactured by symbiotic bacteria which live in our intestines. When refined sugar is taken daily, these bacteria wither and die, and our stock of B vitamins gets very low. Too much sugar makes one sleepy; our ability to calculate and remember is lost.

One lump of sugar in your coffee after a sandwich is enough to turn your stomach into a fermenter. One soda with a hamburger is enough to turn your stomach into a still. Sugar on cereal-whether you buy it already sugared in a box or add it yourself-almost guarantees acid fermentation."

Sugar destroys your immune system, feeds cancer cells, and reduces the body's ability to defend against bacterial infection, sugar interferes with the body's absorption of calcium and magnesium, it raises the level of neurotransmitters: dopamine, serotonin, and norepinephrine; sugar causes hypoglycemia, premature aging, and can lead to alcoholism. Sugar causes tooth decay, leads to obesity, increases the risk of Crohn's disease and ulcerative colitis. Sugar can cause gastric or duodenal ulcers; it can cause arthritis and many more health issues.

Rebounding

66Movement is a medicine for creating change in person's physical, emotional, and mental states. 99

Carol Welch

"Rebounding is an extremely easy exercise in which all that's basically required is a slight up-and-down bouncing to continuously and aggressively clean the body's defense system of waste matter... As little as five or six minutes a day can be of immeasurable value."

Harvey Diamond, Author, *Fit for Life*

Rebounding is my favorite morning ritual — I love it beyond words! As quoted by NASA, exercise on a rebounder or mini trampoline is, *"the most efficient and effective exercise yet devised by man."* It is an excellent, non-impact, aerobic exercise gained by bouncing on a mini-trampoline.

The benefits of exercising on a mini trampoline are astonishing and have been promoted significantly within the last decade. In rebounding, you reach a weightless state at the top of each bounce. As you land, you experience twice the force of gravity, which provides excellent benefits to your muscles, cells, and lymph system.

As we've discussed, the lymphatic system is a crucial wellness system for your body. When waste accumulates and becomes stagnant in this system, individual cells and the systems they are a part of stop functioning as well, leading to illness and disease. It is responsible for getting rid of carcinogens, nitrogenous waste, pathogens, heavy metals, natural waste, and other toxins. Because the lymphatic system has no heart to motivate circulation, practices like exercise, dry brushing and rebounding are crucial parts of a health routine. Rebounding provides the muscular contraction, gravitational pressure, and internal massage to lymph ducts that you need to keep your lymph system healthy.

When you rebound, blood from your arteries can begin reaching the cells that have been cut off by stagnation. The motion, pressure, and exercise encourage your lymph and blood to cycle through your system several times, picking up toxins and delivering food to help your body function at its best.

While I understood the benefits of rebounding, my body didn't agree with it. When I tried a friend's high quality rebounder, I immediately felt a huge difference. My cheap rebounder was actually doing more damage than good. Some mini trampolines cost less than $100, but the surface of these inexpensive models can be unstable and allow too much recoil too quickly which can throw your ankles, knees, and hips out of alignment. I am not endorsing any particular brand however I have tried them all: $50 dollars ones, $350 ones and $700 dollars models. The more you pay, the better quality you get. I had decided to invest in the $700 dollar one because I felt the most benefits to my health from that particular rebounder. I've had it for a few years now and it is still in perfect shape. I love it!

Rebounding is one of the major therapies in our *Health Mastery Retreat*. It is crucial to keep your lymph system moving, especially while cleansing and detoxing.

Happy rebounding my friends!

Yoga

I have been practicing and teaching yoga for the past 7 years and the benefits of this ancient practice are endless. Yoga has been gaining popularity in many domains of the western world. Such disparate people as doctors, vegans, psychologists, and celebrities frequently endorse yoga. More than just a fad, yoga has existed for a millennia, and aims to connect the mind, body and spirit. By hitching your breath and mind to your body, you can achieve numerous physical and spiritual benefits.

The most common form of yoga in the west is *hatha yoga*, which focuses on the physical side of things. By helping flush out invading viruses such as the cold and flu viruses and stimulating the exit of other toxins, it helps lighten the load on your immune system. It uses acupressure points to help encourage this flushing out process. Your immune system can be compromised by stress and fatigue, and yoga provides regular exercise which helps combat these detractors. The discipline provided by a yoga practice may help you to keep to a regular exercise routine and motivate you to make valuable changes in the rest of your life.

Yoga further aids the immune system by improving overall circulation, improving lung health by encouraging controlled deep breathing, clearing mucous from the lungs and sinuses, stimulating internal organ function-ing, and soothing the nervous system. Particular poses or *asanas* can provide more specific benefits. For exam-ple, practiced regularly the Tortoise Posture helps stimu-lates the thymus, therefore increasing the production of antibodies which helps you fight off infection.

I highly recommend you start practicing yoga as one of the healing treatments on your way to health!

Detox

66You can set yourself up to be sick, or you can choose to stay well. 99

Wayne Dyer

Detoxing is even more important than killing Lyme on your healing journey. Every organ and every cell in your body, from your heart to your brain, your lungs, your liver, and your nervous system consumes fuel, such as the food you ingest, to operate efficiently. After using this fuel every cell and every organ in your body produces metabolic waste. Your own body produces metabolic waste daily not to mention that Lyme produces neurotoxins that poison your body and makes you sick.

When your body functions at its peak performance, this waste material is eliminated from your body on a regular basis as fecal matter from your bowel, urine from your kidneys, bile from your liver and gallbladder, sweat from your skin, carbon dioxide from your lungs, and on a cellular level; waste from your blood is eliminated by your lymphatic system.

There have been over 100,000 new chemicals developed since World War 2 and less than 2% of them have been studied for safety. We constantly assimilate toxins from our direct exposure to them; from consuming processed and non-organic food, and from drinking contaminated water to breathing polluted air. Did you know that in the average ten-minute shower, the average human absorbs the same amount of chlorine as if you drank 20 gallons of tap water?! It has also been declared that there is no water to be found anywhere on the planet anymore that does not contain industrial wastes and highly toxic, carcinogenic, mutagenic and disease- causing chemicals, including toxic residues from over 10, 000 different pharmaceutical drugs.

The good news is… most of the healing modalities we have covered above are major detox therapies: high plant-based vegan diet, Bowel Cleanse, Coffee Enemas, Parasites clean up, Dental clean up, Mercury Amalgams removal, Cavitations clean up , Kidney Cleanse, Liver/ Gall Bladder Flush, Juice Fast/Cleanse, Hyperthermia, Contrast showers, Dry skin brushing, Oil Pulling therapy, Heliotherapy, and Rebounding.

I believe all chronic diseases can be cured with a combination of detoxification, alkalizing the body, deep breathing exercise, sweating in the sun, drinking vegetables and herbal juices, following a vegan diet and living an overall healthy lifestyle. There are quite a number of patients, with Lyme disease, Fibromyalgia, Cancer and other chronic diseases, who have recovered based on my coaching and using natural treatments.

Dr. Robert Morse has been practicing medicine for nearly 40 years, and uses simple detoxification methods including a raw vegan diet to help cure people. His core belief is in the ability of the human body to completely recover from any disease. The naturopath has used these methods to treat over 100,000 people who have found relief from a huge variety of diseases including diabetes, candida, kidney stones, fibromyalgia, lupus, Lyme, chronic fatigue, autism, MS, Parkinson's, HIV/AIDS, insomnia, migraines, heart conditions, and cancer.

The regeneration will happen on a cellular level when prompted through the appropriate use of fasting, cleansing, detoxing, and consuming raw living foods. Most people have never tried to fast or detox, and continue to consume highly acidic meals every time they eat. Imagine putting the wrong kind of fuel in a car and expecting it to run perfectly: how long do you think that will last? As debris builds up in different parts of the car it becomes less efficient until it finally breaks down. Unlike a car, the human body can fix itself. Detoxing and fasting gives your body the break that it needs in order to repair itself.

Detox, detox, detox! Go re-read all of the lifestyle suggestions in the chapters above and I promise if you apply them as though your life depends on it, your body will be able to reverse any degenerative condition!

Natural Environment

We have talked already about your skin being the largest organ of your body as well as one of the major detoxification organs. Whatever you apply to your skin gets absorbed into your blood stream instantly. That is why it is so important to avoid all kinds of conventional body lotions, baby oils, deodorants, sprays, etc. They are full of toxic chemicals. Your body is trying so hard to get rid of the metabolic waste and toxic elements you ingest with your food, with the air you breathe, and with the water you drink; why add more toxins?

Personally, my favorite body moisturizer is coconut oil. I apply it all over my body and my face. My skin looks and feels nice and soft. I also apply coconut oil as a lip balm. Coconut oil has tons of benefits and zero chemicals. It's really the best choice for you.

What about your clothing? Your skin actually breathes and eliminates toxins through sweat; it can't be sealed shut! Synthetic fibers like polyester, nylon, Lycra® and spandex don't breathe. They literally suffocate your skin and don't let the toxins out. It is very important to wear natural organic clothes such as organic cotton, silk, wool, and linen.

How about the cleaning supplies for your home? The chemicals that are in them are literally killing you! As I have already stated, over 75, 000 new synthetic chemicals have been developed since WW2 and less than 2% of them have been tested for toxicity. Many are known to cause cancer, neurological dysfunctions, birth defects, and damage all major organs including the liver, kidneys, and brain. Most of these supposedly harmless cleaners and personal care items are extremely toxic. Some are even lethal!

Here are some household chemicals and items that are particularly hazardous. They deserve special mention because their effects can be so debilitating, but they are frequently overlooked.

Commercials have many convinced that **air fresheners** are the only clean smell available, but the way they work is actually very dangerous. Most of them work by blocking and deadening your nasal passages and nerves so that you can no longer smell well enough to notice the bad smells. Many of these "fresheners" use formaldehyde, a toxic carcinogen, and phenol, which is linked to hives, convulsions, circulatory collapse, comas, and death.

Many **cleaning chemicals** are selected because of their intensity, but they make your environment more dangerous instead of clean and safe. **Ammonia** damages your eyes, respiratory tract, and skin, while **bleach** is a corrosive chemical that hurts you in the same way. Mixing ammonia and bleach creates deadly fumes. **Mold and mildew cleaners** can contain sodium hypochlorite (which is corrosive and increases fluid in the lungs) and formaldehyde (like air fresheners). **Antibacterial cleaners** may use triclosan which leads to liver damage when absorbed through the skin.

Carpet and upholstery shampoos have many toxic substances, including perchlorethylene, a nervous system irritant and carcinogen, and ammonium hydroxide, which, like bleach and ammonia, damage your eyes, respiratory tract, and skin. **Furniture Polish** uses phenol (like air fresheners) and nitrobenzene which can be absorbed through the skin to increase toxicity. Furniture polish is a hazardous, flammable material that causes skin and lung cancer. **Car wash and car polish** contain petroleum distillates, which are also associated with skin and lung cancer, as well as fatal amounts of fluid in the lungs.

Pesticides contain dimpylate (diazinon), which is highly toxic. It impairs the central nervous system. They may also contain chlorinate hydrocarbons, which some suspect are carcinogens that are stored in your fatty tissue and assault the nervous system over time. The lungs absorb organophosphates, which are extremely dangerous if you can smell them; which means you've already inhaled them.

Dishwasher detergents, which you would think would be carefully vetted for safety, actually contain chlorine, while **drain cleaners** include a toxic cocktail of lye, hydrochloric acid, and trichloroethane, which together wreak havoc on your digestive and nervous systems. Lye can famously burn your skin, eyes, esophagus, and stomach, and is used to dissolve road kill that is dumped in landfills (imagine what it can do to humans!). Hydrochloric acid damages your skin, eyes, kidneys, liver, and digestive tract, and trichloroethane irritates your eyes and skin and can function as a depressant in your nervous system. **Oven cleaners** also contain lye.

Laundry products can use sodium or calcium hypocrite (a skin and eye irritant), hypochlorite bleach, a corrosive chemical, which burns your skin, eyes and respiratory tract. **Toilet bowl cleaners** may also contain hydrochloric acid (like other drain cleaners) and hypochlorite bleach. When hypochlorite bleach interacts with other chemicals, it can form chlorine fumes that are deadly to humans. **Lice shampoo** is made with lindane, which causes vomiting, convulsions, and circulatory collapse, when inhaled, ingested, or absorbed. It has also been linked to liver damage, stillbirths, birth defects, and cancer.

Many of these "cleaners" include mysterious **fragrances.** The formulas for these fragrances are considered trade secrets, so companies do not disclose the ingredients. An independent review by the National Institute of Occupational Safety and Health found that 1/3 of the substances used in the industry are toxic. Often added to laundry detergents and fabric softeners, these fragrances can cause respiratory irritation, headache, sneezing, and watery eyes. On the bottle, they are simply labeled as "fragrance", so if you see this label it may be something to avoid.

In the kitchen, many of the objects we use to prepare and store food can be dangerous. **Nonstick cookware** uses Polytetrafluoroethylene (PTFE) to prevent food from sticking to the surface of the Teflon. Though this is a time saver, PTFE releases toxic gasses once heated up, which means that every use increases the risk of cancer, organ failure, damage to your reproductive system, and many other ill effects. To reduce risk, cook at lower levels of heat. This strategy does not eliminate risk, so try using other types of pans made of glass, stainless steel, or cast iron. Use cooking oil to reduce the stickiness, and be careful to avoid burning food so that it sticks to the pan. You may also try baking or steaming food; effective strategies for low-calorie, healthy meals.

BPA used in **Plastic Bottles** is notoriously dangerous. By mimicking your hormones, BPA can severely damage your endocrine system. Disposable bottles are probably the worst offenders, because they leak more chemicals (especially when left out in the heat). The bottles allow bacteria to spawn, and the water they contain is not even regulated to the same degree as tap water. Finally, disposable water bottles are simply wasteful: a year's supply for the US requires more than a million barrels of oil. Switching to BPA-free, reusable water bottles is a good move for you *and* the environment.

And NEVER use antiperspirants! Antiperspirants block the sweat glands, preventing sweat from leaving the body. They are extremely effective. Most antiperspirants contain Aluminum Zirconium, and parabens. The sweat your body and skin produce is the elimination of toxins, and if you block it, you are pushing all these toxins back into your tissue.

There are many alternatives to conventional cleaning products. You can buy most of the natural products at the health food stores or even make some yourself. I personally use pure castile soap as a face, hand, and body wash. I make my own bathroom and kitchen cleaner by simply mixing water, vinegar, and some essential oils. You can find all the needed information online about how to make your own household cleaners.

Positivity,
Laughter Therapy

*66A good laugh and a long sleep are the best cures
in the doctor's book. 99*

Irish Proverb

While many of the suggestions in the previous chapters would require some or even a lot of work and changes on your part, this chapter is pure pleasure.

Laughter is a natural gift; a way to show and share our happiness. It lets us feel alive and empowered, and brings us closer to others. Laughter or humor therapy utilizes this natural physiological process, designed by nature to help alleviate stress and discomfort.

The power of laughter to heal our bodies is being discovered over and over across the world. In the film *The Secret*, a woman says she had cured herself of cancer by watching comedies and seeing herself in great health. Norman Cousins healed himself from deadly disease and a massive coronary attack by using nutritional and emotional support protocol of his own design including laughter therapy.

In his book, *Anatomy of an Illness*, the UN peace prize medal winner describes both the gloomy prognosis supplied by the doctors and his recovery. Diagnosed with ankylosing spondylitis, a degenerative disease which causes collagen to break down, Cousins defied doctors and left the hospital. In 1965, they predicted he would die within a few months, but he survived until 1990. Cousins left the hospital almost completely paralyzed, and moved to a hotel room, where he consumed megadoses of vitamin C and a continuous diet of funny movies and other media. He continuously improved until he could move his arms and legs again, and finally returned to his full time job.

And don't forget to limit your time in front of the TV! Watching televised news has been scientifically and medically proven to reduce the ability of your immune system to fight diseases. I have not watched any TV in years and do not have any desire to. You can put on a nice movie, such as a comedy, but stay away from propaganda and mental and emotional violence!

Bad attitudes, negative thoughts, low self-esteem, and playing victim cause diseases! Be positive, love yourself and love your life!

Spiritual Healing

66Just as a candle cannot burn without fire, men cannot live without a spiritual life. 99

Buddha

I was going to finish this book by titling the last chapter, "Positivity and Laughter Therapy" when something interesting happened. My hiking buddy Kevin sent me a brief message that he had an interesting story to tell me about some girl and her spontaneous healing from Lyme. I was more than intrigued, I was eager to hear this story.

I met with Kevin the very next day and he told me that he had just returned from Canada from a spiritual journey retreat. There was a young woman there who was very sick with Lyme disease. When she arrived to the retreat she was extremely weak and had a whole bag of medications to control her symptoms. By the end of the retreat she said that she has not eaten anything for the whole duration of the journey and that she felt Kundalini energy rising in her spine and her symptoms were gone! She felt healed!

I was so touched by this story that I wanted to meet this girl immediately. Kevin connected us and in a few days I flew to New York to meet Tamara. I can confirm that Tamara is a healthy and vibrant young lady with an abundant amount of energy; you could never tell she was chronically ill with Lyme disease. Tamara was shooting her documentary on this horrible disease and she got to interview me for it when we met. Ultimately, it was a win-win for both of us in meeting one another and getting the opportunity to share our stories with each other.

There is no way that I can claim that I am some kind of spiritual guru or master. I do meditate and practice yoga. I pray and practice gratitude. However I would not be able to include a chapter on spiritual healing on my own since I know very little and I have a long way to go. I believe it was meant to be that I met Tamara. She is a perfect example of spiritual awakening and healing and this is her story:

Kundalini Awakening

by Tamara Balsamides

"A silent war was waged against me. One going on inside my own body. My friend just told me yesterday, how healthy I look, how shiny my hair is. I show few symptoms, unless in a total relapse. Then it's blatantly obvious something is wrong; a trip to the bathroom is a struggle. But at that point I'm too sick to even think about company, so no-one really sees what my life has been reduced to.

At my worst, I can't breathe, and I'm severely depressed. Ten years ago I was a vibrant, active mother of two. When graduating from high school I'd already been on my own for two years. I supported myself by waitressing full-time, and graduated with honors from Rutgers with a Psychology degree. Soon after, I met the man of my dreams and slowly etched out quite a wonderful life for myself. There was no need for medical insurance, as I'd never spent a day in the hospital, other than when I was born. I remember being seventeen, walking down a tree-lined street with my then best friend, the one who helped me weather the storms telling her, 'This will play out one of two ways. Either I'll have the most wonderful life, and all my pain is behind me, or, this is just a warm up.' In comparison, my family struggles were a cakewalk.

One afternoon ten years ago, I woke with what I thought was the flu, and a mild one at that. As mentioned mine was an active life raising two small, beautiful girls, (the loves of my life), had a dog, and the loveliest husband in the world. Every weekend we had free, we spent in a park or camping; that is how I connect with God. Because of this Tom proposed to me in one.

After three days of this flu, I'm no better, in fact, much worse. The doctor's thinking was early bronchitis and placed me on antibiotics which worsened my condition. The mood swings were severe and I felt distinctly worse from mere hours earlier. And now, out of nowhere, I felt like the weight of my life was too much to bear, and earlier I was perfectly fine. The pain was unremitting - it felt like there was a spike slowly being wedged into the base of my brain, coupled with migraines, constant nausea, constant dizziness, night sweats, and crippling insomnia. I dropped fifteen pounds and looked like the walking dead, my complexion was ghostly pale with black circles. Most days I couldn't lift my head off the pillow, as I'd get too dizzy. Quite literally I couldn't maintain my own balance. I was having scary cognitive problems, mispronunciation, and an inability to recall simple words like 'cat'. I knew the words, but I couldn't spit it out. I leaned over from my bed into my nightstand and in that split second forgot what I was looking for. There was no frame of reference for this nightmare I was about to descend into. I had babies to take care of.

Tom had to half carry me in to the doctor's office because I now had this funny shuffle walk, and the exertion it required to walk from the car, twenty or thirty steps, to the doctor's office, left me breathless, dizzy and crying. The doctor found nothing in the blood work. But told us my blood pressure was so low I'd have coded in the ER. 'Go home and drink some water with salt in it. And continue the antibiotics.' Did I mention, three weeks earlier being rushed to the hospital, by my husband, with welts from head to toe following days of rashes? What was wrong with me?

I don't know how many doctors I was naive enough to put my faith in over the last ten years. Actually twenty plus years. Since I was in college my health was slowly declining. Knee, hip problems, mitral valve prolapse, very serious flu's every year, mastitis three times. MS was suspected, and since nothing was found in the blood work I learned to just navigate around these annoyances. It wasn't until that 'flu' ten years ago that the walls came crashing down.

Dutifully, each doctor's program I followed until it was obvious something was still terribly wrong. I've been rushed to the hospital three times; I've had Pneumonia four times, and have been wheel-chaired on and off airplanes, to my extreme embarrassment. My hormonal system and immune system still aren't working correctly. There isn't a body system unaffected. I had MVP and a heart murmur. I had a very rapid pulse and low blood pressure, which no one could explain. I had unexplained Mono and Pleurisy. I've been diagnosed with Hypothyroidism, Osteopenia, Chronic fatigue syndrome, Fibromyalgia, Celiac disease, and Lupus. I've had good days over the last ten years, but never normal ones. If my diet is pristine-organic, lots of vegetables, if I don't drink, or smoke, avoid sugar, sleep a minimum of 9 hours a night, rest a lot, (and still usually need a nap), I have a half day of energy. In ten years, I've never been able to do anything more strenuous than walking or Yoga. The palpitations start, my heart races, it skips beats, I feel ill, and it can push me into a relapse for days.

My Herbal Medicine degree has kept this illness at bay, coupled with very high doses of Vitamin C. Ten years later, I read Vitamin C is actually one of the natural cures, and I'd been inadvertently treating this illness all along. I experimented a lot, and found huge success with castor oil packs, and seaweed baths. My sole criterion was to keep the infections at bay. As far as the seaweed baths went, I learned later that they break up biofilms, the protective barriers around the Lyme dis-

ease spirochete. The biggest problem I encountered was my immune systems inability to fend off the smallest infection, which was a disaster with two small girls in school. Ten to thirty grams of Vitamin C daily kept me alive. Because my immune system markers were so low, I was diagnosed with Lupus. The relapses, during exposure to infection, were like bouts of the flu. Imagine having the flu, every two to three weeks, interminably. Every time Tom or one of the girls came home with the sniffles I was crippled – every single time.

Once, Tom had to race me to the hospital because I couldn't stay conscious due to vomiting and diarrhea at the same time. Literally, I'd get pale, sweaty, and pass out. Quite funny in hindsight, the police pulled us over as we were racing; he took one look at me, and directed us to the hospital. The problem is I, in my thirties, had no frame of reference for endless illness. It's not like I can't take pain. I delivered my last baby sans pain killers. This illness in its chronic stage is as debilitating as Congestive Heart Disease, which is why it has the highest suicide rate. You never get a break. And during all this endless, pointless suffering, no one believes you.

Here I was, at severe onset, a thirty one year old woman, with a one year old baby to care for, and a four year old. The only help I had was my sister, who saved my life, almost single-handedly – her and Tom. We had to hire nannies, then full-time help, a housecleaner. I couldn't unload the dishwasher from the exertion without stopping three times to catch my breath, or walk up one flight of stairs.

Yet, the emotional destruction trumps the physical. The worst assault wasn't feeling abandoned, or neglected, or even seeing the damage this had done to my children. Lyme disease also stole from me my third child I desperately wanted and destroyed my sexual relationship with my husband. I've not only not been unaided by my community, but have had to contend with vicious rumors going around in my town. What if my children hear this? Don't they have enough to deal with?

Additionally, family snickering behind my back, or openly calling me a hypochondriac. One family member, in front of my children, commented that it'd have been cheaper if I'd died. In hindsight I don't know how I made it through this time.

The worst part for me is the 'Chump' part. Because even though it's caused immeasurable suffering on my behalf, I've been played. I've been played by a system that didn't give me adequate testing. That told me unequivocally that I did not have this illness, not once, but twice. The standard two-tiered LD test has a forty percent effectiveness rating. Compare this to the AID's test, which is ninety-nine percent effective. I went to two specialists for this specific disease and countless others, when I did my research and knew what this was. One specialist said I definitively did not have this illness and withheld the fact that the PCR test she ran had a thirty percent effectiveness rating. I lost another three years, and thousands of dollars.

So have you guessed it yet? Drum roll, please... Yes, Lyme disease. So now that I have a diagnosis smooth sailing, right? Not so fast. When you can get antibiotics, due to insurance restrictions, based on IDSA guidelines, they leave you incredibly ill. Whatever progress I'd made over the past ten years is down the toilet because in killing these spirochetes, they release neurotoxins and once again you feel like the walking dead. Since starting treatment, I've spent weeks bedridden, unable at times to sit up. I had to treat aggressively with antibiotics for over a year. In the meantime I get to hope that I don't have permanent damage to my heart or brain.

My dear friend, sick with the same illness, has a PIC line out her arm, and IV antibiotics. (My insurance company won't give it to me), because the IDSA has ruled that Chronic Lyme disease doesn't exist. I suppose I'm a medical anomaly, as are thousands of others. Other life threatening infections, such as TB, and AIDS have open-ended treatment protocols. The IDSA has set a two week limit on the antibiotic treatment for Lymies.

My above mentioned friend also has all three kids under the age of ten infected, and her husband. She can't rest, and recover; she's got to get them treated. An entire family disabled and no one understands it, or lends the smallest hand to help her. That's the tipping point. Where's the community rallying around us? This is unconscionable, and unheard of in any other life-threatening condition. I can't imagine shrugging off someone with a Cancer diagnosis. Both illnesses are deadly, the difference is LD takes much longer, while you are isolated, and in many cases, denied treatment. It affects every body system so you never truly get a break. I read a quote once. She says, 'I've been diagnosed with Cancer twice, and Lyme disease. I'd swap Lyme disease for both Cancers any day.' This is not to diminish the severity or importance of Cancer, only trying to place Lyme disease in the proper context.

We fight and fight and fight, to get diagnosed and then realize the marathon has only just begun. I'm not so angry with the doctor's because I believe in my heart most of them had my best intentions at heart. The IDSA members responsible for setting Lyme disease guidelines - I'm livid with. Quite frankly, they have blood on their hands. A conservative estimate from the CDC reported that there are 200,000 new cases a year, five times that of AIDS, in the whole United States. The latest reports, the newest estimates are that it's epidemic in my part of the country. I consider myself bright, well-educated, and at least a quarter of a million dollars later, I finally have an answer only because a dear friend got her diagnosis. We'd been going back and forth for years comparing notes, and I knew we had the same thing. So one month, I spent another thousand dollars, out of pocket, to see my third specialist. He explained to me that the more chronic this infection is, the more the antibodies glob onto the bacteria, and there's none left circulating in your blood system to be picked up by even the best blood work. The spirochete sequesters itself in the tissue, and the evidence of this is known, and yet tests keep being done looking for it in the blood. So if the IDSA says there's no such thing as chronic Lyme disease, and gives out a test looking in the wrong place, they are right!

Lyme disease is the most obvious answer given my locale, (it's an epidemic in NJ), my outside activity, living surrounded by trees, having dogs, and my reaction to the antibiotic. How was this missed? Why was I diagnosed with everything but the most obvious illness? My very strong reaction to the antibiotic I was administered in the beginning of the illness should have been another clue to the doctors. Lyme disease is the only disease that makes you much sicker once you start antibiotics. Thankfully I had some resources financially. If I hadn't, I would not still be here.

We're currently fifty thousand dollars in medical debt. My oldest child was tested and guess what? She also has it. Her medical costs are another $1,500, for the first month! As does my littlest one. Lyme disease is reported as more virulent than syphilis. It is sexually and congenitally transferred. It just never ends. Well, that's unless you are someone powerful, such as George Bush and New Jersey Governor, Christie Todd Whitman. They both had Lyme disease, but somehow got adequate testing and prompt treatment. I guess we weren't important enough.

So whose war is this? And, in whose best interest was it to patent it in 1980? And in God's name, if there's no cover-up, why are the few doctors trying to test this illness losing their medical licenses? Why, are the two bands most highly specific for chronic Lyme disease, NOT on the standard testing? If they had been, my life would have taken a completely different trajectory. Since I can't change that, all I want is the testing to change; and others to not have to die.

I tell people I caught the wrong illness. I caught the one that's a big scam. It wasn't well known in the US before 1970, then the people that re-discovered it, patented it. Since then it has become more virulent and paired with co-infections. I had three co-infections. Alone these are deadly. One of them is related to Malaria. Imagine having Syphilis and Malaria, and additional infections all at the same time. And yet one doctor I saw tried to tell me I was creating this so I could get out of housework.

Documentaries are being filmed, mine being one of them, A Ticking Time Bomb. I needed to channel my outrage into a positive forum. People are dying, massive productivity is lost. One madman with chronic Lyme went on a killing spree. It is a brain infection after all. Group suicides are happening as people can no longer cope, and don't want to continue to drain their family's already depleted resources. They see no way out.

In July of 2011, I treated myself to a one week sacred tour of the Canadian Rockies with David Wilcock. I'd been reading his books about ascension and the upcoming earth changes and felt compelled to go. I saved up for the trip, and spent a week in the most pristine surroundings. Our home base was this family owned chateau staffed with the loveliest, most caring people. Every day we visited a sacred site and David lectured at night.

I was 10 months into my LD treatment, and had what I thought was a LD attack on the plane. This had happened before, as the altitude kills off the LD organism, and the ensuing neurotoxin release is a nightmare. I became sweaty, nauseous, my head was pounding, especially the back of the neck, by the occipital bone. I got very dizzy, but thank God that this time I didn't vomit. This was terrifying, as a woman traveling alone, to a different country, knowing no one when I arrived. Literally I couldn't walk off the plane to get through customs. Too weak to wheel my luggage, and despite my embarrassment, I had to stop every 10-15 steps. Once in the bathroom, I just wept. I was white as a ghost, and had no choice but to just surrender, again. I was getting quite good at this. My human side protested, saying I've been sick over 20 years, I'm alone; I just want one good thing. So, I surrendered. I said God, I am in your hands, and I accept this. I don't know why, but I accept it. Eventually, I did feel a little better, and found a quiet place to nap and regain my strength. Later I met up with the group.

That night we drove to Hanmer Springs, with purported healing waters. The next evening we checked into our chateau. That day we spent at Lake Louise. I write in my journal that I'm blissed out; I weep for joy at the majesty of the Lake. It feels as if a very special connection has been bridged. A year later, I learn that it's a very high energetic spot and an etheric retreat for ascended masters.

At the Chateau our host tells us that she has energies that work in the house to bring about healing, and that if so inclined, we can pray for a healing. Despite my reservations, I do pray that night. It can't hurt. The next day I've slept six hours and have energy, normally I need at least ten. The day after that, I sleep only six again but awake with no fatigue. I'm feeling very well, not a familiar feeling, so it was quite distinct. I also am losing my appetite, and crying one minute from bliss, the next from releasing pain. The following day I'm down to four hours of sleep, no fatigue, can't eat a thing, literally. It's quite odd to sit with people eating and not partake in this ancient ritual. It felt so uncomfortable, sensing that I was making them uncomfortable, that I soon stopped joining them at mealtime. I was running circles around people. One man commented I was the energizer bunny, having no idea what that meant to someone with the energy of a person with congestive heart failure. I was also feeling very, very, strong energy running up and down my spine - like butterflies on speed.

By the third day I feel so well that I go off my medications. My regimen had been two antibiotics for the LD, an anti-malarial for a co-infection, and thyroid medicine, and bags of supplements. My suitcase was full of seaweed for the baths I'd needed to take every night, gluten free food for the Celiac disease from the LD, castor packs for the pain. I needed none of it, and photographed a plate full of supplements and medications I'd have needed without this healing.

By the fourth day, I'm sleeping three hours a night. I forgot to mention that I'm blissed out all the time. I can feel the energy in the trees; I'm seeing sacred geometry in the heavens. My dreams are nothing like regular dreams; I'm in sacred, angelic places, often getting healings. There's a feeling of a distinct connection to God, and humanity. In the next moment I'm weeping, shedding some pain that's been buried forever. But it felt cleansing, healing, and there was no fear. I just felt. Previously, the fear thing was huge for me, given I couldn't walk up a flight of stairs or fold laundry. I literally had no fear. It was completely obvious to me that any time I was scared or fearful I wasn't in a place of love. Since all I could feel was love, this fear thing felt wrong and alien, versus the other way around that I had been living. All that I wanted to do was be in nature, and listen to beautiful music. There was nothing to do, nowhere to go, only this space to just be. It was all perfect, as was I. The energy surges became more profound, even painful, and I found the only relief I got was to lie on the ground, connect my whole body with the earth. I later learned I was grounding the energy to the Earth.

So, after a week of this I return home. I've learned that there's a name for this glorious experience. I've had a spontaneous Kundalini Awakening. The energy that lies dormant in all our spines had for me become activated. What do I attribute this to? My years of meditation? My surrender to a higher power during this illness? Or was it my dogged determination to heal my wounds, feel my pain, and forgive all. Possibly, the healing springs, or the energy in the house, or the etheric retreat. I think it's all the above. I set the spiritual groundwork, and was compelled to be in an energetic place that met the needs of this energetic healing. You see the force of Kundalini is so strong that illness cannot co-exist in the body.

My girls got a new mom the day I returned home. The one they should have had all along. I now could play tennis and bowl, and swim, and do all the things I loved with them. I was elated and plugged in!

As far as my body was concerned, I didn't eat a meal for nine whole days. I still evacuated every day, which tells me how hard my body was working at repairing the seat of my immune system. It was a month before I needed more than four hours of sleep a night. I now have two distinct sets of dreams. The ones before 2 AM are of a spiritual nature. I'm in heavenly places learning or being healed, in the presence of Angels or Ascended Masters. The dreams after that time are the regular linear ones with people and storylines.

The first thing I did was to call my doctor and ask for a prescription for a whole panel of blood work. She asked me why, and when I told her about the healing she congratulated me. Sure enough, all clear, including the thyroid. The only thing on there was a high viral load - I've had cold sores my entire life. Interesting.

At a year later I'm almost completely healthy. I am enjoying family time and have devoted myself to raising awareness of the Lyme disease epidemic, and helping those still suffering. I've produced a documentary in the hopes of bringing about awareness. Adversity for me isn't a bad thing. For me, that's my limited human judgment not being able to see the big picture. The rewards of overcoming LD are immeasurable for me personally, and for our family. My girls have seen adversity, strength, resilience and healing. They've learned compassion, and understanding. Our family is stronger now than ever."

Final Thoughts

Congratulations! You have made a first step towards your healing by reading this book. Now you have a choice – you can choose to apply all the principles you have learned in this book and heal yourself, or you can doubt them. You can choose to become a warrior or remain a victim. You can choose to follow the mainstream and let them brainwash you with the propaganda, or you can choose to step up. It is up to you if you get well or remain *dis-eased*. It is up to you, my friend!

Make a decision right now to take full responsibility for your health and heal yourself. Make a decision to change and never look back. Make a decision to be a warrior and not a victim. Make a decision to live your life to the fullest and make those around you happy. Make a decision to tell your loved ones you love them before it's too late. Make a decision, my friend, right here right now and life will never be the same again!

God Bless,

Katrina Starzhynskaya

Acknowledgements

First off, I would like to thank Meghan Snell, my tireless editor, for her dedication and hard work. Without you Meghan, this book would not have happened.

A special thank you to Olga Matunina for going with me to Montreal. Thank you Dr. Peter Veniez for all your help and your healing. Thank you to my friend Brigitte for your support. Thank you Laney Tant for widening my world about natural healing and for your healing sessions. Thank you Lai San Leung for your help, care, and your healing—of course. Thank you to my friend Larisa for helping out with autohemotherapy when no one else would perform it.

Remember, *nothing* is incurable! Get **Empowered!** Get **Well!**

Notes

PART 1
MY JOURNEY

It is ALL in YOUR HEAD!

1. Excerpt from Dr. Jemsek's remarks to the NC medical board in 2006.

What is Lyme disease?

1. http://ocmotherwarrior.com/lyme-definition/
2. http://www.crazylyme.com/p/what-is-chronic-lyme-disease.html
3. http://myremedi.com

Does Chronic Lyme Even Exist?

1. http://ocmotherwarrior.com/lyme-definition/
2. http://www.crazylyme.com/p/what-is-chronic-lyme-disease.html
3. http://rense.com/general69/lyme.htm

Is Lyme disease a Biological Warfare?

1. http://www.umm.edu
2. *Lab 257* by Michael C. Carroll

Welcome to the Club!

1. www.mdjunction.com

Taking Full Responsibility for your Health

1. *Insights into Lyme Disease Treatment*, Connie Strasheim, p.138

Medical Prognosis

1. *Creating Health* by Deepak Chopra, MD
2. *20 Powerful Steps to a Healthier Life*, Dr. Schulze, p. 50 (online version here https://herbdocblog.com/bookview/12/)

Absolute Faith

1. Dr. Lee Cowden, MD (*Insights into Lyme Disease Treatment*, Connie Strasheim, p.168)
2. *The Cure for all Diseases*, Hulda Clark, p.1
3. *http://www.merriam-webster.com/medical/jarischherxheimer+reaction*
4. *http://www.dorlands.com*

Supplements,   Antibiotics – Cure or Poison?

1. Dr. Ingo D.E. Woitzel, MD (*Insights into Lyme Disease Treatment*, Connie Strasheim, p.188)
2. Ronald Whitmont, MD (*Insights into Lyme Disease Treatment*, Connie Strasheim, p.207)

Cowden Protocol

1. www.bionatus.com/nutramedix
2. Dr. Lee Cowden, MD (Insights into Lyme Disease Treatment, Connie Strasheim, p.148)
3. *Insights into Lyme Disease Treatment*, Connie Strasheim, p.151

Buhner's Protocol

1. *Healing Lyme: Natural Healing and Prevention of Lyme Borreliosis and Its Coinfections* by Stephen Harrod Buhner

Dr. Zhang and Modern Chinese Medicine

1. http://www.sinomedresearch.org/

Two Feathers Healing Formula

1. http://www.healingformula.net/

Acupuncture plus Apitherapy

1. http://www.apitherapy.org/about-apitherapy/what-is-apitherapy/

Dr. Whitmont, Homeopathy

1. *Insights into Lyme Disease Treatment*, Connie Strasheim, p.205

Autohemotherapy

1. http://www.altmeds.com/autohemotherapy/description

Advanced Cell Training

1. http://advancedcelltraining.com/
2. http://www.time.com/time/

My Experience with a Rife Machine

1. http://blog.frequencyfoundation.com/
2. http://frequencyfoundation.com/forms/Photo-Analysis.pdf
3. http://rifemachinebuilder.com/3.html
4. *The Cancer Cure That Worked: 50 Years of Suppression* by Barry Lynes

MMS – Miracle Mineral Solution

1. http://wildalchemist.blogspot.com/2009/02/mms-de-mystified-sodium-chlorite.html

"Gu Syndrome" - Demons of the Body & Mind

1. http://www.classicalpearls.org/

Chemtrails: What in the world are they spraying?

1. http://www.geoengineeringwatch.org/category/chemtrails/
2. http://chemtrailsdisease.com

Brain Fog and How to Deal with It

1. http://naturopathconnect.com/articles/brain-fog-causes/

2. http://www.myadrenalfatigue.com/brain-fog-relief

3. http://www.earthclinic.com

Family/Friends Drama

1. (Geri Fosseen, Director, of the Iowa Lyme Disease Foundation, Melissa Kaplan's Chronic Neuroimmune Diseases Information on CFS, FM, MCS, Lyme Disease, Thyroid, and more)

Letters from those with "Invisible" Illnesses

1. Susan Williams, PublicHealthAlert.org via http://wholelifeliving.ning.com/profiles/blogs/10-commandments-for

Success Stories

1. Heather Levine, http://www.ladderbridges.com/

2. Marissa Cassella, Story written exclusively for this book.

Mindset to Achieve Outstanding Health

2. *Unleash the Power Within* by Tony Robbins

PART 2
MASTER PRINCIPLES OF VIBRANT HEALTH

1. Dr. Ginger Savely, DNP (*Insights into Lyme Disease Treatment*, Connie Strasheim, p.120)

2. *How to Get Well*, Dr. Paavo Airola p.17

3. PowerPoint presentation by Dr. Richard Horowitz at the Lyme Disease Conference, San Diego, CA May 6, 2012

4. champ.htm

5. Dr. Steven Bock, MD (*Insights into Lyme Disease Treatment*, Connie Strasheim, p.74)

6. *Unleash the Power Within* by Tony Robbins

Diet Equals Health!

1. *Super Immunity*, Dr. Joel Fuhrman, MD, p.1

2. *20 Powerful Steps to a Healthier Life*, Dr. Schulze, p.75 (online version here https://herbdocblog.com/book-view/12/)

3. *The China Study: The Most Comprehensive Study of Nutrition Ever Conducted and the Startling Implications for Diet, Weight Loss, and Long-term Health* by Dr. T. Colin Campbell

4. Dr. John McDougallhttp://veganstreams.com/plant-based-diet-healing-diabetes-heart-disease-osteoporosis-planet/

5. Neal D. Barnard, M.D., President, Physicians Committee for Responsible Medicine, Washington, D.C

6. *Vegan Nutrition: Pure and Simple* by Dr. Michael Klaper

7. William C. Roberts, M.D., editor of *The American Journal of Cardiology*

8. Arthur Schopenhauer quote, http://www.quotationspage.com/quote/25832.html

9. *20 Powerful Steps to a Healthier Life*, Dr. Schulze, p.73

Gerson Therapy

1. *The Gerson Therapy: The Proven Nutritional Program for Cancer and Other Illnesses* by Charlotte Gerson and Morton Walker, D.P.M.

2. http://gerson.org/gerpress/the-gerson-therapy/

Body Cleansing

1. http://www.publichealthalert.org/Articles/victoriabowmann/Cleansing%20Neurotoxin%20Overload.html

Bowel Cleanse

1. http://www.crystalinks.com/egyptmedicine.html

2. http://www.publichealthalert.org/Articles/victoriabowmann/Cleansing%20Neurotoxin%20Overload.html

3. http://coffee-enema.ca/coffeeenemaprocedure.htm

Parasite Cleanse

1 .http://www.publichealthalert.org/Articles/victoriabowmann/Cleansing%20Neurotoxin%20Overload.html

2. http://prairielymelight.com/?p=138

3. http://curezone.com/cleanse/parasites/default.asp

Dental Clean Up/Mercury Amalgams

1. http://www.bostondentalwellness.com/mercury-freenatural.html

2. http://proliberty.com/observer//20091008.html

3. http://www.shirleys-wellness-cafe.com/amalgam.htm

4. http://www.cdchealth.com/mercuryamalgamdanger.html

5. http://www.healthfirstdental.com/articles/what-is-biological-dentistry.aspx

6. M.M. Van Benschoten, "Acupoint Energetics of Mercury Toxicity and

7. Amalgam Removal with Case Studies," *American Journal of Acupuncture*, Vol.

8. 22, No. 3, 1994, pp. 251-262.

Danger of Root Canals, Cavitations

1. http://westonaprice.org

2. http://articles.mercola.com/sites/articles/archive/2012/02/18/dangers-of-root-canaled-teeth.aspx

3. http://www.davidicke.com/forum/archive/index.php/t-201283.html

4. http://articles.mercola.com/sites/articles/archive/2012/02/18/dangers-of-root-canaled-teeth.aspx

5. http://www.toxicteeth.org

Kidney Cleanse

1. http://www.how-to-boost-your-immune-system.com/kidney-cleanse.html

2. http://eatinghealthy.blogspot.com/2007/06/kidney-maintenance-protecting-your.html

3. https://herbdocblog.com/article/Answer/bladder-tumor=gone/

Liver/Gallbladder Cleanse, Flush

1. http://www.globalhealingcenter.com/natural-health/liver-cleanse-foods/

2. *The Amazing Liver & Gallbladder Flush* by Andreas Moritz

3. http://www.drclark.net

4. *The Cure for All Advanced Cancers*, Hulda Clark, p.562

Juice Fast

1. http://www.freedomyou.com/juice_fasting_freedomyou.aspx

2. http://www.drfosteressentials.com

Hyperthermia

1. http://www.steinerhealth.org/health/fever-therapy/

2. http://www.the-natural-path.com/hyperthermia.html

3. Bastyr College Natural Health Clinic: http://www.bastyrcenter.org/

4. http://www.aromaspas.com/category/aromaspas___parts.health_benefits/

Contrast Showers/Hydrotherapy

1. http://www.outofstress.com/contrast-shower-benefits/

2. http://www.naturopathicthoughts.com/2008/12/benefits-of-contrast-showers.html

Dry Skin Brushing

1. http://www.holistichealthlibrary.com/dry-skin-brushing-and-the-lymph-system/

Oil Pulling Therapy

1. http://www.naturalnews.com/025578_oil_pulling_health.html

2. http://earthclinic.com/Remedies/oil_pulling.html

3. http://www.jonbarron.org/detox/nl110404/oil-pulling-strong-immunity

4. http://oilpulling.com

Heliotherapy

1. http://sunlightenment.com/heliotherapy-benefits-of-sunbathing/

2. http://www.sciencemuseum.org.uk/broughttolife/techniques/heliotherapy.aspx

3. http://www.naturalnews.com/030598_vitamin_D_Institute_of_Medicine.htm

4. http://www.naturalnews.com/031560_vitamin_D_cancer.html

5. http://www.naturalnews.com/rr-sunlight.html

6. http://www.naturalnews.com/032815_sunscreen_chemicals.html

7. *More Natural "Cures" Revealed*, Kevin Trudeau, p.64-66

Stop Your Sugar Addiction NOW!

1. http://articles.mercola.com/sites/articles/archive/2010/04/20/sugar-dangers.aspx#_edn1

2. Dr. William Coda Martin   http://www.globalhealingcenter.com/sugar-problem/refined-sugar-the-sweetest-poison-of-all

3. *Sugar Blues* by William Dufty

Rebounding

1. http://tudecidesmedia.com/health-rebounding-p3699-128.htm

2. http://health101.org/products_rebounder.htm

3. http://juice4life.com.mx/benefits_of_rebounding/rebounding_detoxification_effect.htm

Yoga

1. http://yogamodern.com/categories/science/77-surprising-health-benefits-of-yoga-2/

2. http://blog.gaiam.com/blog/author/sadienardini/

3. http://yoga-health-benefits.blogspot.com/2009/06/yoga-for-immune-system.html

Detox

1. http://www.atlanteanconspiracy.com/2011/09/cure-for-everything-fasting-detox-and.html

Natural Environment

1. https://www.achooallergy.com/blog/dangerous-household-chemicals/Default.asp

2. http://www.organicconsumers.org/articles/article_279.cf

3. http://www.alternet.org/story/141196/10_dangerous_household_products_you_should_never_use_again

Positivity, Laughter Therapy

1. http://www.cancercenter.com/complementary-alternative-medicine/laughter-therapy.cfm

2. http://www.thesecret.tv

3. http://www.healingcancernaturally.com/laughter-is-medicine.html

4. *Anatomy of an Illness* by Norman Cousins

Kundalini Awakening by Tamara Balsamides

1. Tamara Balsamides, Story written exclusively for this book.